The Epilepsies

95

The Epilepsies
MODERN DIAGNOSIS AND TREATMENT

John M. Sutherland
MD (Glasg) FRCP (Edin) FRACP
Honorary Consultant Neurologist, Royal Brisbane Hospital
Visiting Consultant Neurologist, Toowoomba General Hospital
Honorary Reader in Neurology, University of Queensland

Mervyn J. Eadie
MD PhD (Qland) FRACP
Professor of Clinical Neurology and Neuropharmacology
University of Queensland

FOREWORD BY
Professor Henry Miller
MD (Durh) FRCP DPM
Late Vice-Chancellor, University of Newcastle upon Tyne

THIRD EDITION

CHURCHILL LIVINGSTONE
EDINBURGH LONDON AND NEW YORK 1980

CHURCHILL LIVINGSTONE
Medical Division of the Longman Group Limited

Distributed in the United States of America by
Churchill Livingstone Inc., 19 West 44th Street,
New York, N.Y. 10036, and by associated companies,
branches and representatives throughout the world.

First edition 1969
Second edition 1974
Spanish edition 1976
Third edition 1980

ISBN 0 443 02184 8

British Library Cataloguing in Publication Data
Sutherland, John Mackay
    The epilepsies. – 3rd ed.
    1. Epilepsy
    I. Title   II. Eadie, Mervyn J
    616.8'53   RC372   80–40030

Printed in Singapore by Singapore Offset Printing Pte Ltd

Foreword

Few physicians escape responsibility for the management of patients with epilepsy. Except in a small group of very resistant cases the attacks can usually be fairly well controlled with the very effective anticonvulsant drugs now available. Indeed many patients can achieve complete freedom from fits for the small price of scrupulously maintained medication. Nevertheless epilepsy is not in general treated as well as it should and might be. This is not because treatment is hazardous, complicated or uncomfortable, but because it demands time and patience on the parts of both patient and doctor. Some doctors feel they have done all that is required when they hand the patient a bottle of phenobarbitone tablets. Some patients find a regular routine of morning and evening tablets too troublesome to observe: they furnish most of the cases of status epilepticus. In fact no two patients are alike. Epilepsy is a disorder of infinite variety, in which unhurried therapeutic experiment and careful individual adjustment of dosage with appropriate drugs pay handsome dividends.

Dr Sutherland and Dr Tait have written an up-to-date and realistic account of epilepsy, based on personal interest and vast clinical experience, that goes far beyond the best of textbook presentations. Not only will it stimulate professional interest in the condition, but indirectly it will bring the benefits of more effective treatment to thousands of patients.

Newcastle, 1969   H.M.

Preface to the Third Edition

In this edition we have again attempted to present a contemporary account of The Epilepsies for senior students, house officers, practitioners and others wishing a short, practical book on the subject.

Since the last edition, significant advances have occurred in investigatory methods and in drug therapy. Previously, the timing of major investigations such as angiography or air encephalography called for some nicety of judgement since if performed too early an underlying disease process, if present, might not be apparent. It was understandably difficult in some instances to have these tests repeated at a later time should this prove desirable. This problem has been obviated by the advent of the safe, non-invasive and painless technique of computerised tomography of the brain. The current methods of investigating a patient presenting with epilepsy are included in the appropriate chapter.

Anticonvulsant drug therapy has now achieved a more rational basis. Several drugs formerly in use have been largely superseded by more effective preparations and indications for the use of the various anticonvulsants have become more clearly delineated. The ability to estimate plasma drug levels has placed the dosage and frequency of administration of anticonvulsants on a scientific rather than on an empirical basis. These matters and the interaction of anticonvulsants are discussed in the chapters on treatment and anticonvulsant drug therapy which have been extensively revised.

References for further reading have been expanded and up-dated. No attempt has been made to furnish a complete list of references but we again acknowledge our indebtedness to the many authors whose work has influenced our views and our practice.

We dedicate this edition to the late Professor Henry Miller, Newcastle upon Tyne, England, and to the late Dr Howard Tait, Brisbane, Australia.

Brisbane, 1980   J.M.S.
                                                                              M.J.E.

Preface to the First Edition

Cassius: But soft, I pray you: What! did Caesar swound?
Casca: He fell down in the market-place, and foamed at the mouth, and was speechless.
Brutus: 'T is very like: he hath the falling sickness.

Shakespeare: *Julius Caesar*
Act 1, Scene 2

Epilepsy (the 'sacred disease', the 'falling sickness') is a common condition and it has been estimated that some four or five individuals in every 1000 of the population suffer from some form of epilepsy. Despite this, it is our impression that many undergraduates and some practitioners find the epilepsies a confusing subject. This has possibly been occasioned by the numerous classifications and synonymous terms encountered in the literature, brought about by two separate approaches to the subject, the clinical on the one hand, and the pathological on the other.

Because we feel that most practitioners demand information and an understanding of the clinical aspects of epilepsy—the measures to employ when confronted with the practical issues of diagnosis and management—we have orientated this book to clinical and practical aspects rather than to pathophysiological and theoretical ones. Although no claim is made for originality, and we gladly acknowledge the debt we owe our own teachers and the many authors who have influenced our thinking, the views expressed are also based on our personal experience and practice. No attempt has been made to furnish a bibliography. It is hoped that in the pages which follow the reader will find a readily understood account of epilepsy which will prove of help to senior medical students and to practitioners who may wish to read a current account of this subject.

The authors would like to express their thanks to their clinical teachers and the many authors who have influenced their opinions, and to Dr P. A. Tod for Figures 26, 27, 28 and 29. We are indebted to the Editor, *The Medical Journal of Australia,* for permission to reproduce Figures 8 and 30, and thank Dr M. J. Eadie for carefully reading the proofs.

We wish to thank Professor Henry Miller who so kindly agreed to write the foreword, and our publishers for their help, forbearance and courtesy throughout the preparation of this book.

Brisbane, 1969   J.M.S.
                                                                   H.T.

Contents

1

General considerations and classification

As the term 'The Epilepsies' suggests, there is no single disease 'epilepsy'. Rather, there is a group of disorders, the epilepsies, which appear to involve similar pathophysiological mechanisms but which develop in different anatomical regions of the brain, have different aetiologies and are associated with different electroencephalographic appearances. For convenience, however, throughout this book the word 'epilepsy' will be used as a synonym for 'The Epilepsies'.

Epilepsy is best regarded as a symptom, due to a commonly occuring type of brain dysfunction. Other types of disturbed brain function of course exist. When confronted with a patient who gives a history of one or more brief episodes of disturbed brain function the clinician has to consider the following possibilities:

1. Epilepsy
2. Consequences of disturbed cerebral blood flow
    a. physiological e.g. vasovagal syncope
    b. pathological e.g. transient ischaemic attacks, 'drop' attacks of vertebro-basilar arterial insufficiency
3. Consequences of altered blood composition e.g. hypoglycaemia, drugs
4. Brain pathology e.g. brain stem lesions, tumors within the ventricular system
5. Narcolepsy–cataplexy syndrome
6. Psychiatric disorders e.g. hysteria, catatonia
7. Malingering

EPILEPSY

It is difficult to better Hughlings Jackson's century old definition, 'A convulsion is but a symptom, and implies only that there is an occasional, an excessive and a disorderly discharge of nerve tissue . . .' Such a definition includes under the diagnosis of epilepsy the situation of the individual who has had but one seizure and who may never take another. Because of the social and medico-legal implications which customarily attend a diagnosis of epilepsy, it may therefore be preferable to employ a rather less embracing definition such as the following: epilepsy is a condition characterised by recurrent discrete episodes, primarily of cerebral origin, in which there is a disturbance of movement, sensation, behaviour, perception and/or consciousness.

Unfortunately, this definition excludes seizures which in their clinical features are identical with epileptic seizures, but which are due to recognisable extracranial causes such as hypoglycaemia, uraemia or eclampsia. The clinician seeing a patient with a seizure may well have to look outside the nervous system to determine the cause of that seizure. *It is therefore proposed to define and regard epilepsy as a symptom due to excessive temporary neuronal discharging which results from intracranial or extracranial causes: epilepsy is characterised by discrete episodes, which tend to be recurrent, in which there is a disturbance of movement, sensation, behaviour, perception and/or consciousness.*

The word 'fit', as used in ordinary speech, has various meanings. Although it may be a synonym for 'seizure', the latter term will be preferred in the present text.

The nature of epilepsy
The precise mechanisms involved in producing the excessive neuronal discharges of epilepsy remain incompletely understood. It would seem that there are a number of possible mechanisms whereby a group of neurons may become hyperexcitable and prone to excessive discharging.

1. *Altered neuronal membrane potentials* Neurons are kept in a state of excitability by virtue of ionic concentration gradients across their cell membranes. The concentration of Na^+ ions within neurons is considerably lower than the Na^+ concentration in extracellular fluid, whereas intracellular K^+ ion concentrations are very much higher than extracellular K^+ concentrations. The net effect of these concentration gradients of cations and anions across the neuronal cell membrane is to keep the cell membrane in a polarised condition, the interior of the cell being at a negative potential relative to the exterior. Disease-induced alterations in extracellular Na^+ (or Ca^{++}) concentrations may alter neuronal excitability throughout the nervous system. If extracellular Na^+ or Ca^{++} concentration falls relative to intracellular concentration (as in Addison's disease or hypoparathyroidism) the potential difference across neuronal cell membranes may fall toward the threshold at which a self-propagating action potential develops. Thus neurons become hyperexcitable and the risk of epilepsy increases. It is not known whether local cerebral disease can alter neuronal

cell membrane potentials in the region of the site of pathology.

2. *Altered synaptic transmission* Excitability of the post-synaptic cell membrane of neurons may be altered by the release of synaptic transmitter chemicals into the synaptic cleft. Thus at appropriate synapses acetylcholine release has an excitatory effect, while at other synapses gamma aminobutyric acid (GABA) acts as an inhibitory transmitter. Deficiency of pyridoxal phosphate, which catalyses the synthesis of GABA, can decrease GABA-mediated inhibition in certain pathways to such an extent that these pathways become hyperexcitable enough to cause clinical epilepsy. It is not known whether local cerebral disease can cause epilepsy by altering synaptic transmitter activity, though the possibility exists. Certain drugs which prevent epilepsy alter the concentrations of synaptic transmitter molecules, including GABA, serotonin and noradrenaline.

3. *Altered activity of inhibitory neuronal pools* Particularly at a cerebral cortical level, many groups of neurons appear to act mainly by inhibiting other neurons. If local cerebral disease develops it may damage an inhibitory neuronal pool. If so the neurons innervated by this inhibitory pool may become denervated, and therefore disinhibited and hyperexcitable. It is thought that such local disinhibition is the mechanism whereby local brain damage due to trauma, infection, ischaemia or neoplasm may cause epilepsy.

4. *Altered generalised neuronal excitability* As well as the factors discussed above which increase brain excitability by known mechanisms, other factors exist which may increase neuronal excitability diffusely via biochemical or bioelectrical mechanisms which are inadequately understood. Such factors include pyrexia, hypoxia, overhydration, alkalosis, withdrawal of barbiturates, diffuse cerebral disease (e.g. neurolipoidosis) and various toxins. Possibly some of these factors (e.g. overhydration, alkalosis) alter neuronal cell membrane potentials, and others may alter the activities of synaptic transmitter chemicals, but the detailed mechanisms of action are not established. Such factors increase neuronal excitability diffusely. If there are collections of neurons with a pre-existing heightened excitability, such diffusely acting factors are likely to bring these more excitable neurons to the point of epileptic discharging before other neurons reach this threshold.

5. *Altered epileptic threshold of the brain* Even when none of the above factors capable of producing epilepsy is known to be present, every living brain can still be made sufficiently hyperexcitable to produce an epileptic seizure if exposed to an electrical flux of sufficient intensity. The critical intensity varies from person to person. Thus the concept arises of an intrinsic seizure threshold of the brain, and this

concept can be extended to take in more than electrically-induced seizures. Seizure threshold is probably determined by peculiarities of individual brain biochemical and bioelectrical functioning, but the natures of these pecularities are totally unknown at present.

Except in relation to electrically-induced seizures the existence of a seizure threshold is not readily proven. However, the concept helps explain why a provoking factor may produce epilepsy in one brain but not in another, although otherwise the brains seem identical. The individual seizure threshold appears to be a factor related to the production of epilepsy above and beyond those more tangible factors discussed above. Sometimes a low seizure threshold appears to be inherited, in that some genetically determined mechanism results in an increased susceptibility to epilepsy in members of a family. A very low seizure threshold may be exceeded without demonstrable cause. A somewhat higher threshold may be exceeded only if brain excitability is heightened when the individual brain is exposed to the action of factors such as pyrexia, hypoglycaemia or drug withdrawal. When intracranial lesions (e.g. those resulting from trauma, infection, vascular disease or neoplasia) are present, the individual seizure threshold may determine whether or not epilepsy occurs.

In terms of the concept of seizure threshold, epilepsy is a relative rather than an absolute type of abnormality. There is, indeed, a continuum ranging from normal individuals (who have never had a spontaneous seizure and would have one only if exposed to a rather extreme stimulus e.g. a convulsant drug or a high voltage electrical shock), through people with seemingly normal brains who have seizures apparently precipitated by physical upsets (e.g. fatigue, fever, alcoholism), by particular afferent stimuli (e.g. flickering lights, specific sound frequencies, sudden movements) or by emotional stress, to those who have attacks without demonstrable provocation in the presence of brain disease, and even in the absence of detectable brain abnormality.

More than one of the factors discussed above may be present at the same time to determine the occurence of any given seizure. Thus a group of neurons may be relatively disinhibited because the relevant inhibitory neuronal pool is damaged by disease. However, this group of neurons may not become sufficiently hyperexcitable to produce a clinical seizure until neuron excitability generally is increased by fever or by hypoglycaemia.

The behaviour of epileptic discharges
The manner in which an epileptic discharge expresses itself clinically depends on the part of the brain in which the excessive discharge

begins and the parts through which it spreads (Fig. 1). Discharges originating in the upper brain stem (mesodiencephalic reticular formation: centrencephalic system) project diffusely and simultaneously to the whole cerebrum; such a primarily generalised discharge is associated with impaired consciousness with or without bilateral motor events. An epileptic discharge commencing in an area of the cerebral cortex may remain localised; or, initiated locally, the discharge may spread locally to activate adjacent cortical neurones; or initiated locally, the discharge may spread by corticothalamic pathways to activate the mesodiencephalic mechanisms in the deep central grey matter of the upper brain stem, resulting in turn in a

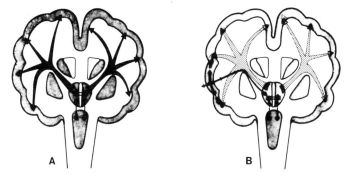

Fig. 1a and **b** Diagrams showing simultaneous and symmetrical spread of a generalised epileptic discharge from certain thalamic and mesencephalic regions to the whole cerebral cortex (Fig. 1a), and local cortical spread of a partial epileptic discharge (Fig. 1b) with subsequent spread of the discharge to the thalamus and then possible secondary generalisation activating the whole cortex.

further diffuse projection of the discharge to the whole cerebrum (a secondarily generalised discharge). The local discharge in the cortex evokes the usual manifestations of the function of that part of the cortex in which the discharge begins, and through which it spreads. If the discharge becomes secondarily generalised, the typical manifestations of a generalised epileptic discharge (*viz.* impaired consciousness with or without bilateral motor events) becomes superimposed on the manifestations of the local cortical discharge. Thus a focal motor (Jacksonian) seizure may remain localised to the fingers of one hand; the seizure may spread locally to involve the hand, forearm, arm, and perhaps the leg on the same side; or the local manifestation of the cortical discharge may be followed by a generalised convulsion and loss of consciousness identical with the generalised convulsion and loss of consciousness resulting from a primarily generalised discharge originating in the mesodiencephalic reticular formation.

Table 1   Classification of epilepsy based on aetiology

---

1. *Idiopathic (primary or constitutional) epilepsy*
   No apparent cause
   Characterised clinically by:
   Major seizures (grand mal)
   Minor seizures (absences: petit mal)
                   (myoclonic seizures)
                   (akinetic seizures)

2. *Symptomatic (secondary) epilepsy)*
   a. Due to intracranial causes
   b. Due to extracranial causes
      Characterised clinically by:
      Focal cortical symptoms
      Focal cortical symptoms preceding a major seizure (grand mal)
      Myoclonic seizures

If a focal cortical discharge originates in a silent area of the brain (e.g. frontal lobes or non-dominant temporal lobe), the initial discharge may not occasion any obvious symptoms. If this discharge should spread to the mesodiencephalic reticular formation the patient may present with the clinical picture of a generalised discharge without the preliminary symptoms which suggest a discharge beginning in the cerebral cortex.

Classification of epilepsy

From the foregoing it will be apparent that some patients have epilepsy from a known recognisable cause (e.g. head injury, cerebral neoplasm, hypoglycaemia, drug withdrawal), while other patients have seizures for no demonstrable reason. It is, therefore, possible to classify epilepsy on an aetiological basis as indicated in Table 1.

More recently, the International League against Epilepsy has proposed a classification which is gaining wide acceptance. This classification is based on seizure pattern interpreted in terms of the probable site of seizure origin in the brain. There is a subsequent correlation of this primary criterion with the aetiology of the epilepsy. The full classification is too extensive for convenient clinical application but it can be abbreviated as in Table 2. In this classi-fication, *Generalised seizures* are characterised by the following features:

1. The abnormal discharge originates in or close to the mesodien-cephalic reticular formation and almost instantly projects widely or diffusely throughout the cerebrum.

2. The surface electroencephalogram shows diffuse synchronous and symmetrical discharges of spike and slow wave form.

3. Clinically, consciousness is impaired from the outset and

bilateral motor events may occur; both disturbances are of varying severity and duration so that attacks may range from transient lapses of consciousness (absences; petit mal), through lapses of consciousness with varying amounts of bilateral clonic jerking (myoclonic absences) to tonic, clonic and tonic-becoming clonic seizures (grand mal).

4. Aetiologically, the excessive discharging of the mesodiencephalic reticular formation is often related to genetic factors which render the system unstable. Rather less often, it may be due to structural pathology or chemical causes. It is possible that only, or mainly, the hereditary types of generalised epilepsy begin in the mesodiencephalic reticular formation. In primarily generalised epilepsy of acquired aetiology, the excessive discharge may originate outside the mesodiencephalic reticular formation but spreads to this region so rapidly that only the subsequent generalised projection of the discharge can be detected clinically or on surface electroencephalography. In such instances depth electrode recording may indicate the true local origin of the excessive discharge.

Partial seizures have the following features:

1. The excessive discharge occurs from a group of neurons

Table 2   Classification of epilepsy adapted from classification proposed by International League against Epilepsy (1969)

1. *Generalised seizures*
   Bilateral symmetrical seizures without local onset;
   clinically:
   a. Absences
   b. Bilateral myoclonus
   c. Infantile spasms
   d. Clonic seizures
   e. Tonic seizures
   f. Tonic-clonic seizures
   g. Akinetic seizures

2. *Partial seizures*
   Seizures beginning locally with:
   a. Elementary symptomatology
      motor
      sensory
      autonomic
   b. Complex symptomatology
      impaired consciousness
      complex hallucinations
      affective symptoms
      automatism
   c. Partial seizures developing into generalised tonic-clonic seizures

3. *Unclassifiable seizures*
   Seizures which cannot be classified because of incomplete data

anywhere in the brain other than the mesodiencephalic system. The discharge may remain localised, spread locally or spread widely to involve the mesodiencephalic system which may then be activated resulting in a generalised seizure secondary to the primary cortical event.

2. In the surface electroencephalogram discharges begin locally although they may subsequently become bilateral or diffuse.

3. Clinically, the events depend on the site of the local discharge and whether it remains localised or spreads locally, or spreads widely to involve the mesodiencephalic reticular formation. The manifestations are protean.

4. Aetiologically, partial epilepsy is always due to local brain pathology (though this pathology may occasionally be hereditary e.g. tuberose sclerosis).

The *local brain pathology* responsible for epilepsy may be classified according to the patient's age:

Childhood—adolescence
Cerebral birth injury, anoxic or otherwise.
Congenital and developmental anomalies including arteriovenous malformation.
Sequelae to meningitis or encephalopathy.

Adult life under 50 years
Head injury.
Mesial temporal lobe sclerosis, often due to earlier brain hypoxia.
Cerebral tumours, often primary.
Arteriovenous malformation.

Adult life over 50 years
Cerebrovascular occlusive disease.
Cerebral tumours, primary or metastatic.
Cerebral atrophy.

As mentioned earlier, there are a number of extracranial causes of epilepsy. If the brain is structurally normal, these causes are likely to bring the mechanisms involved in primarily generalised epilepsy to the pitch of hyperexcitability at which seizures occur before the rest of the brain is so activated. Therefore these extracranial causes of epilepsy find expression as primarily generalised seizures. However, if there is a local abnormality in the cortex, the extracranial cause of epilepsy may bring local cortical neurons to the point of discharge before the mesodiencephalic reticular formation reaches it seizure threshold. In this cause, the extracranial cause of epilepsy will produce partial seizures.

Extracranial causes of epilepsy include:

Anoxic disturbance
e.g., heart or respiratory arrest.

Endocrine disorder
e.g., hypoglycaemia: hypocalcaemia.

Renal disease
e.g., uraemia.

Pregnancy
e.g., eclampsia.

Poisons and toxins
e.g., alcohol, lead, chlorinated hydrocarbons (insecticides), barbiturate withdrawal.

In general, the International League's (1969) Classification of Epilepsy will be followed in this book, but equivalent terms from the aetiological classification will be given where appropriate. The relationship between the two classifications is shown in Table 3. It should be noted that focal (symptomatic) seizures and partial seizures are largely synonymous. However, primary (idiopathic) epilepsy is not quite equivalent to generalised epilepsy in that the latter term includes not only primary seizures but bilateral seizures due to intracranial and extracranial disease processes.

Relative frequency of different types of epilepsy
Gastaut *et al.* (1976) have provided an analysis of the types of seizures found in 6000 of their patients. An abbreviated version of their figures provides some idea of the relative frequency of the different types of epilepsy among sufferers from the disorder. The type of seizure could not be classified in almost 24 per cent of the series. Generalised epilepsy occurred in 38 per cent of the classifiable cases, (including 28 per cent of the classifiable cases who had tonic-clonic fits, 9 per cent who had absences, 4 per cent who had idiopathic and 9 per cent who had acquired myoclonic seizures, with some patients having more than one type of seizure). Partial epilepsy occurred in 62 per cent of the classifiable cases (10 per cent with seizures with an elementary symptomatology, 40 per cent with complex symptomatology and 13

Table 3   The relationship between the two classifications of epilepsy discussed in the text

Aetiology of epilepsy	Clinical pattern	Onset of epilepsy
Primary (idiopathic)	Petit mal absences	
Primary or symptomatic	Myoclonic seizures	
	Tonic or clonic seizures	*Generalised*
	Tonic→clonic seizures	
Symptomatic	Focal seizures ±	
	Secondary tonic-clonic seizures	*Partial*

per cent with seizures that underwent secondary generalisation). Thus for rough purposes partial epilepsy appeared nearly twice as common as generalised epilepsy.

SUMMARY

1. **Disturbed cerebral function including impairment of consciousness** is likely to be caused by one of the following:

    (i) Epilepsy
    (ii) Disturbed cerebral blood flow ──┬── Physiological
                                          └── Pathological
    (iii) Disorders of blood composition
    (iv) Structural brain disease
    (v) Narcolepsy – cataplexy syndrome
    (vi) Psychogenic disorders
    (vii) Malingering

2. **Epilepsy** is a symptom of excessive neuronal discharging due to a variety of intracranial or extracranial causes.

3. **Neuronal excitability** is influenced by:

    a. Ion concentration gradients across the nerve cell membrane.
    b. Release onto the post-synaptic cell membrane of excitatory and inhibitory substances.
    c. Activity of inhibitory neuronal pools.
    d. Various diffusely acting factors such as pyrexia, overhydration.
    e. Seizure threshold of the brain.

4. The result of an epileptic discharge depends on its site of origin in the brain and its extent of spread within the brain.

Discharge originating in mesodiencephalic
reticular formation⟶diffuse spread
                 through cerebrum

                 impaired consciousness
                    ±
                 bilateral motor events

Discharge originating in
cerebral cortex⟶May remain localised
                May spread locally
                May spread to involve mesodiencephalic system
                ⟶ diffuse spread

5. Classification of epilepsy—two systems:

A

Generalised seizures	**Idiopathic (primary) epilepsy**
Absences	Major seizures (grand mal)
Bilateral myoclonus	Minor seizures
Infantile spasms	Petit mal absence
Clonic seizures	Myoclonic
Tonic seizures	Akinetic
Tonic-clonic seizures	
Akinetic seizures	

B   **Symptomatic**
Partial seizures   **(secondary) epilepsy**

With elementary symptomatology   a. Intracranial causes
With complex symptomatology   b. Extracranial causes
Partial seizures becoming generalised

Unclassifiable

6. Conditions causing or activating epilepsy

Intracranial┬Trauma   **Extracranial**┬Anoxia
          ├Infections   ├Endocrine disorder
          ├Degeneration   ├Toxins
          ├Vascular lesions   ├Poisons
          └Tumour   └Drug withdrawal

7. Relative frequency of various types of epilepsy

Generalised—38 per cent ⎱
Partial   —62 per cent ⎰ of classifiable cases of epilepsy.

FURTHER READING

Gastaut H 1969 Clinical and electroencephalographical classification of epileptic
    seizures. Suppl. Epilepsia 10: 2
Gastaut H, Gastaut J L, Goncalves e Silva G E, Sanchez G R F 1976 Relative
    frequency of different types of epilepsy: a study employing the classification of the
    International League against Epilepsy. Epilepsia 16: 457
Gloor P 1969 Neurophysiological basis of generalised seizures termed centrencephalic.
    In: Gastaut H, Jasper H, Bancaud J, Waltregny A (eds) The physiopathogenesis of
    the epilepsies. Charles C Thomas, Springfield
Jasper H H, Ward A A, Pope A 1969 Basic mechanisms of the epilepsies.
    Little, Brown and Co, Boston
Whitty C W M 1965 A note on the classification of epilepsy. Lancet 1: 99
Williams D 1958 Modern views on the classification of epilepsy. Brit Med J 1: 661
Williams D 1965 The thalamus and epilepsy. Brain 88: 539

2

The clinical features of epilepsy

GENERALISED EPILEPSY
(Including Idiopathic i.e. Primary Epilepsy)

Epileptic discharges which begin in, or rapidly spread into, the mesodiencephalic reticular formation, may then suddenly and synchronously project to the whole cerebrum. If so, in the mildest form of such generalised epilepsy a wave of cortical suppression rapidly follows each discharge, and the seizure that develops is characterised by a brief lapse of consciousness only (an *absence* or *petit mal* seizure). Where cortical inhibition is less efficient the lapse of consciousness may be accompanied by one or several brief bilateral muscle jerks (various patterns of myoclonic seizure). Where there is relatively little cortical inhibition bilateral motor events dominate the clinical picture, though consciousness is still interrupted.

Generalised epilepsy may result in the following clinical types of seizures:

1. Absences.
2. Bilateral myoclonus.
3. Infantile spasms.
4. Clonic seizures.
5. Tonic seizures.
6. Tonic-clonic seizures.
7. Akinetic seizures.

Diagnostic criteria for generalised epilepsy
1. The clinical pattern of the seizure.
2. The age of onset—almost always during the first or second decades of life.
3. Frequently a familial incidence.
4. No abnormal neurological signs in the primary (hereditary) variety.
5. Characteristic electroencephalogram changes commonly present.

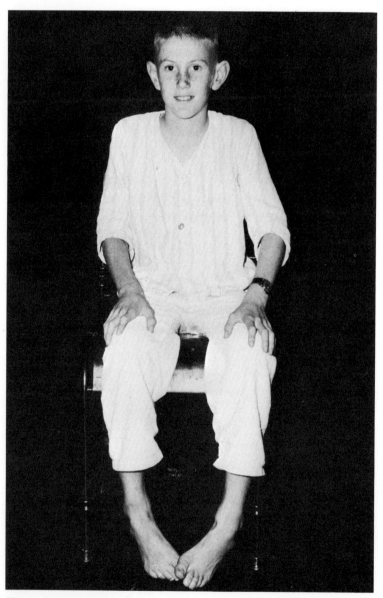

Fig. 2a Petit mal seizure—normal.

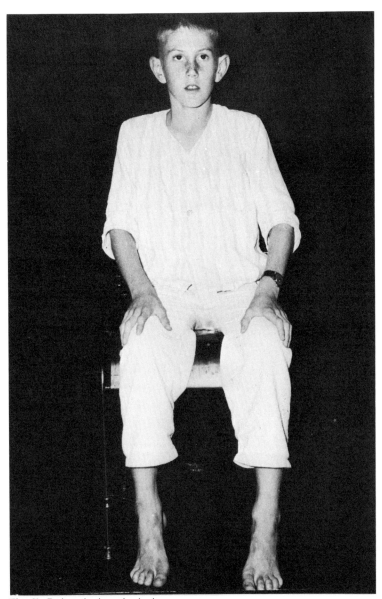

Fig. 2b Petit mal seizure beginning.

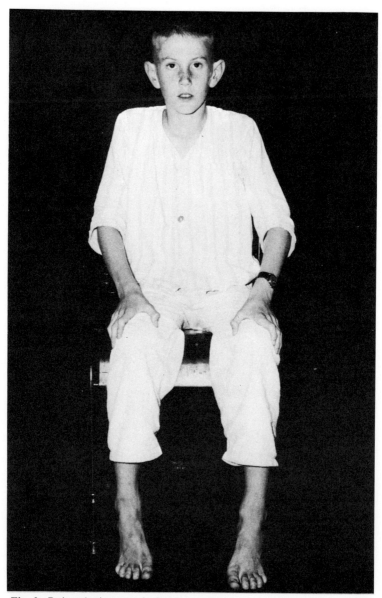

Fig. 2c Petit mal seizure continuing.

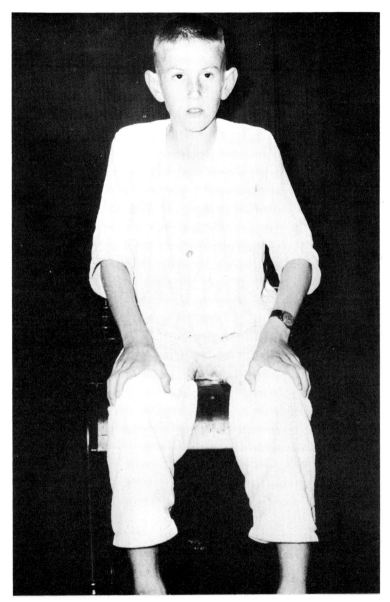

Fig. 2d Petit mal seizure continuing.

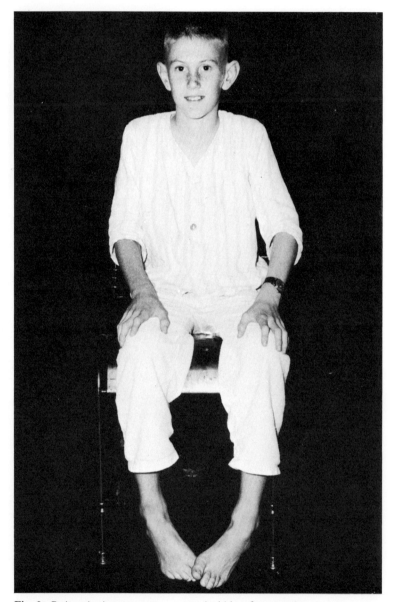

Fig. 2e Petit mal seizure—return to normal within a few seconds.

ABSENCES
(Minor seizures, petit mal)

Absences (or lapse attacks or petit mal seizures) are of short duration, rarely lasting more than a few seconds. In these transient breaks in the continuity of consciousness the patient, usually a child, behaves in the following characteristic manner (Fig. 2):

1. He abruptly ceases whatever he is doing—eating, playing or talking.
2. He may 'stare' ahead or his eyes may roll upwards.
3. For some seconds he is non-responsive, neither speaking nor understanding the spoken work.
4. Thereafter he continues with what he was doing before the attack and may not be aware of the episode.

Such attacks may be very frequent, 10, 20 even 100 occurring daily, and in some instances the abnormal electrical discharges occur almost continually (*absence, benign or petit mal status*), the patient remaining in a relatively confused state.

Absences may occur alone or may be associated with major tonic-clonic (grand mal) seizures of primarily generalised epilepsy.

Unfortunately the term 'petit mal' has been endowed with different meanings. Some employ it to denote purely lapse attacks (absences) as described above; others have included in the term certain myoclonic and akinetic seizures; yet others employ 'petit mal' to denote any seizure short of a generalised convulsion. We restrict the term to denote a particular variety of (idiopathic) generalised epilepsy, commonly of hereditary origin, characterised clinically by absences and electroencephalographically by bursts of bilaterally symmetrical and synchronous 3 Hz spike and slow wave activity occurring at highest voltage in the frontal regions.

Certain patients with *akinetic seizures* and *myoclonic attacks* may have reasonably similar, 2–5 Hz spike and slow wave, or polyspike and slow wave, electroencephalographic changes; hence the term 'petit mal triad' (absences; akinetic seizures; myoclonic attacks). Although these disorders may be hereditary, clinically similar akinetic and myoclonic seizures occur in symptomatic epilepsy and it would be therefore advisable to qualify, for example, the designation myoclonic epilepsy, by indicating whether it was hereditary or acquired in aetiology.

Similarly, minor epileptic seizures clinically suggestive of petit mal absences but lacking the characteristic electroencephalographic changes, may arise from a cortical epileptogenic focus, particularly in a temporal lobe. This is, of course, a variety of partial (symptomatic) epilepsy with a pathological basis. The electroencephalogram will often indicate the focal origin of the seizure. Features helping to distinguish between absence seizures and minor attacks of partial epilepsy of temporal lobe origin are set out in Table 4.

AKINETIC AND MYOCLONIC SEIZURES

Myoclonus is best regarded as a motor expression of a hyperexcitable neuronal system. It can arise at cranial nerve (e.g. facial nerve), spinal cord or brain stem (palatal myoclonus) level but these manifestations are not usually thought of as epileptic. Epileptic myoclonus appears to arise from bilateral discharges originating in or near the mesodiencephalic reticular formation. It is usually manifested as jerking of both upper and/or lower limbs and may be associated with attacks of loss of postural tone (akinetic seizures), or tonic-clonic (major) seizures.

Myoclonic seizures, as already mentioned, may occur in *idiopathic epilepsy* (often associated with electroencephalographic changes rather similar to those of petit mal absences). Similar seizures with bilaterally synchronous high amplitude electroencephalograhic paroxysms of various forms also occur as a manifestation of *acquired epilepsy* in the following circumstances:

Table 4   The differences between idiopathic petit mal absences and minor attacks of partial epilepsy of temporal lobe origin

	Petit mal	Temporal lobe seizure
Age	Childhood–20 years	Any age
Aetiology	Idiopathic—constitutional—hereditary	Secondary to trauma, anoxia, infection, tumour etc.
Frequency of attacks	Numerous or very numerous	Less frequent; often nocturnal and then may not be recognised
Postictal manifestation	Nil	Often some postictal confusion
E.E.G.	Bilaterally synchronous symmetrical 3 Hz spike and slow wave activity	Often a focal discharge in a temporal lobe
Other investigations	Not usually indicated	Desirable—X-ray skull, CT scan ± isotope brain scan ± air encephalogram or angiography
Treatment	ethosuximide clonazepam valproate	Treat cause if possible Drugs: phenytoin primidone carbamazepine sulthiame

1. *Diffuse brain pathology* e.g. lipoidosis, subacute sclerosing encephalitis, tuberose sclerosis (myoclonus sometimes produced by startle e.g. slapping examination couch or clapping hands).
2. *Familial myoclonic epilepsy.* A progressive familial degenerative condition characterised by:
   a. myoclonic and akinetic seizures
   b. major tonic-clonic seizures
   c. extrapyramidal symptoms
   d. cerebellar symptoms
   e. dementia.
3. *Action myoclonus.* A sequel to hypoxic damage or encephalitis.
4. *Infantile spasms* (hypsarrhythmia; West's syndrome).
5. *Lennox–Gastaut syndrome.*
6. *Biochemical disorders* e.g. uraemia, hepatic failure.

Generally, *nocturnal myoclonus*, a sudden myoclonic jerk occurring as the individual is about to fall asleep, is entirely benign and has no clinical or epileptic significance. It can be regarded as being similar in significance to occasional déjà vu experiences in that both are reminders of the potential instability of the normal nervous system.
   Infantile spasms. This particular variety of generalised (symptomatic) epilepsy occurs in infants. There appear to be two aetiological groups.

1. The infantile spasms are possibly related to a delay in the maturation of the cerebrum.
2. The condition is associated with gross cerebral pathologies—e.g. cerebral birth trauma, various types of encephalopathy, tuberose sclerosis, congenital defects.

The onset is generally between three and seven months of age, the initial symptom being brief nodding attacks (often mistaken for petit mal absences), jackknife attacks (in which the body suddenly flexes forwards) or salaam attacks (characterised by upward movement of the arms and then flexion of the trunk). In some instances one leg may extend at the hip, and the spasms are often associated with a cry. These spasms usually occur in clusters several times each day and, as the name 'spasm' or its synonym 'lightning seizure' suggests, they are generally momentary. They occur against a background of restless movements and the majority of affected infants are or become mentally subnormal. Generalised tonic-clonic epileptic seizures may also develop.
   The usual anticonvulsants have little or no effect on infantile spasms, but it is important to recognise this condition since in at least a

proportion of cases, corticotrophin, tetracosactrin or corticosteroids appears to arrest the condition clinically, and this is accompanied by improvement in or even a reversion to normality of the electro-encephalogram. The electroencephalogram is usually characteristic, the name hypsarrhythmia being applied to the abnormality (large amplitude generalised irregular slow waves with sharp waves and spikes arising from multiple foci and often present during sleep when they alternate with periods of low voltage activity).

One variety of infantile spasms appears to be related to some genetically determined state characterised by a greater than usual pyridoxine requirement. In this group there is a dramatic clinical response to the intravenous injection of pyridoxine and this can be followed by oral administration of the vitamin.

The Lennox–Gastaut syndrome. This variety of myoclonic epilepsy, sometimes euphemistically called 'minor motor' epilepsy, tends to begin in childhood, often about the age of four to six years. The disorder is usually of acquired aetiology. There are repeated bilateral myoclonic jerks, sometimes of considerable severity. The child may be thrown to the ground by the violence of the jerks, and may be injured in falling. The epilepsy often interferes with education, and tonic-clonic (grand mal) seizures may develop. The condition does not respond well to anticonvulsants in most instances, and corticotrophin and steroids are not of benefit.

Tonic seizures. These are characterised by the individual's assuming an abnormal posture for seconds or minutes with or without loss of consciousness. Generally there is flexion of the upper limbs and extension of the lower limbs. The condition possibly relates to release of the basal ganglia from cortical control. This type of seizure may occur in intracranial disorders (e.g. encephalitis, birth trauma) or in extracranial disorders (e.g. hypocalcaemia).

TONIC-CLONIC SEIZURES
(Major seizures, grand mal, generalised convulsions)

These are characterised by the following sequence of events:

1. There may sometimes be a prodromal period of irritability and tension lasting for several hours or days.
2. There is no aura in epilepsy originating from the meso-diencephalic reticular formation. The patient usually without warning suddenly loses consciousness, becomes rigid in extension, sometimes with a cry, falls to the ground, may urinate and is apnoeic.
3. After a number of seconds of intense tonic spasm of face, trunk and

limbs, a brief period of interrupted tonus ensues, followed by generalised bilaterally synchronous jerking of face, arms, trunk and legs.

4. These clonic movements gradually become less frequent, less intense and finally cease, leaving the patient comatose and flaccid.

5. Consciousness slowly returns, often with postictal symptoms of confusion, headache and drowsiness.

Tonic-clonic seizures are the most severe expression of generalised epilepsy. Patients who have absences, or myoclonic seizures, may at other times have tonic-clonic seizures. Sometimes myoclonic seizures may increase in frequency over some hours till a generalised tonic-clonic seizure occurs. The secondary generalisation of partial seizures may also lead to bilateral tonic-clonic seizures.

PARTIAL (SYMPTOMATIC) EPILEPSY

The concept that epilepsy can have a focal origin in the brain is not new. Hughlings Jackson in 1888 described seizures produced by lesions of the uncus. As indicated earlier, the initial abnormal electrical discharge in partial epilepsy may remain localised (for example, twitching of a finger may be the sole epileptic manifestation) or it may spread in a variety of ways.

1. The discharge may spread in a sequential manner along a gyrus in a Jacksonian march (for example, from finger to wrist, to forearm, to arm).

2. The discharge may spread centrifugally from the site of origin (for example, adversive turning of the head may follow spread of a discharge to the premotor cortex in a seizure originating in the temporal lobe or frontal lobe.

3. The discharge commencing focally in the cortex may spread along corticothalamic pathways to the diencephalon to activate the deep grey matter of the mesodiencephalic reticular formation with loss of consciousness and the production of a major tonic-clonic seizure by secondary generalisation of the discharge.

The symptomatology of the partial seizure will depend on the site of the abnormal discharge and often constitutes reliable localising evidence. It has been suggested that partial epilepsy may be caused by an abnormal electrical discharge at either end of the corticothalamic axis and that an irritable focus in the diencephalon may discharge by thalamo-cortical pathways to a segment of the cortex. However, for clinical purposes partial epilepsy should equate with symptomatic epilepsy, almost always due to focal cortical pathology. *It is vital to recognise that partial (focal, usually cortical) seizures, have an underlying pathology.* It is, therefore, not sufficient to diagnose epilepsy of focal origin; one must usually be prepared to investigate also the nature of the underlying pathological process which has produced this focal disturbance of brain function. As will be discussed in more detail later, a focal cortical seizure may produce only focal symptoms; such focal symptoms may precede a generalised convulsion; in some instances the patient may not be aware of any focal disturbance preceding his seizure, and it is in such cases that an erroneous clinical diagnosis of generalised (usually idiopathic) epilepsy may be made. It will be apparent that any symptom or sign of disturbed cortical function preceding an apparent generalised seizure very strongly suggests the focal origin and symptomatic nature of the epilepsy. These disturbances of cortical function, whether they be motor, sensory or psychic, preceding a major seizure are often referred to as the aura. In this sense the use of the term 'aura' may be misleading since the aura is the focal or partial seizure preceding the secondarily generalised seizure. If this, however, is appreciated, aura and focal or partial seizure are virtually interchangeable terms.

Focal cortical (partial) seizures may arise from any part of the cortex and can be classified according to their clinical manifestations and site of origin—motor, sensory and so on. In the past, seizures originating from the temporal lobe were described as epileptic equivalents or, because of their frequent psychic content, as psychomotor seizures. In fact the vast majority of seizures with some disturbance of psychic function can be identified with temporal lobe epilepsy, which is itself a variety of partial epilepsy.

Symptoms
Seizures originating in the motor cortex result in clonic, sometimes tonic movements which begin locally in a limb or part of a limb; in the sensory (post-rolandic) parietal cortex, paraesthesiae or more rarely dysaesthesiae may be experienced. Lesions in the occipital cortex produce either negative seizure phenomena (sudden brief impairment of vision in part of or in the whole visual field), or positive phenomena (often unformed visual hallucinations, e.g. flashing lights). If the adjacent temporal lobe is also involved, formed hallucinations may be experienced e.g. a complex scene. Frontal lobe seizures are frequently devoid of focal manifestations, consciousness being lost without warning when the discharge generalises thus suggesting erroneously a clinical diagnosis of generalised (idiopathic) epilepsy. Occasionally seizures with a psychic content have their origin in a frontal lobe.

Although status epilepticus may complicate any form of epilepsy, there appears to be a particular predisposition to this complication of epilepsy in frontal lobe seizures. Seizures originating in the temporal lobe are of particular importance because of their frequency and will therefore be dealt with in greater detail below.

Temporal lobe seizures

These comprise about one third of all epilepsies and the psychic content of the seizures renders them especially susceptible to misdiagnosis.

Causes

The temporal lobe is particularly vulnerable to damage and therefore the production of epileptogenic foci, for the following reasons:

1. *Hippocampal herniation* through the free edge of the tentorium may occur during the birth process or as a result of oedema of the infant's brain. This herniation interferes with the blood supply to the temporal lobe through the anterior and posterior choroidal arteries, with resulting anoxic damage and gliosis (incisural sclerosis; Ammon's horn sclerosis; mesial temporal lobe sclerosis).

2. Parts of the temporal lobe appears to be particularly susceptible to *anoxia* from any cause and also to *hypoglycaemia*.

3. The *acceleration-deceleration head injuries* of adult life not infrequently result in damage to the anterior and inferior aspects of the temporal lobe by the sphenoidal wing.

4. *Infection* from the middle ear and mastoid may spread to involve the temporal lobe.

5. Although *infarcts, neoplasms, harmartomas* and *vascular mal-formations* may affect any part of the brain, such lesions occurring in relation to medial aspects of the temporal lobe seem to have a greater epileptogenic potentiality than similar lesions occurring elsewhere.

Symptoms

The temporal lobe type of partial epilepsy in different persons may give rise to extremely varied patterns of symptoms which can be summarised thus:

Epigastric sensation. This somatic hallucination, a peculiar, usually unpleasant sensation, often described as fear, commencing in the epigastrium and rising up into the chest and throat, is one of the commonest symptoms. It may be associated with sensations in the mouth and lips and involuntary swallowing.

Hallucinations. These may affect perception of smell, taste, hearing, vision and posture (vertigo). Sometimes the visual disturbance is an illusion rather than an hallucination, objects appearing small, distant or distorted. Hallucinations are typically difficult to describe since, because they result from disturbed function, they are often outside the patient's normal experience.

Disturbance of memory. Déjà vu (undue sense of familiarity with unfamiliar environment), jamais vu (feeling of unfamiliarity with known environment), a sensation of time standing still or rushing past, as in panoramic memory, may be all experienced. Sometimes there is forced recall of scenes, words or phrases.

Dreamy states. Feelings of unreality (derealisation or depersonalisation) are also experienced.

Primary automatism. Primary automatism should be distinguished from secondary automatism which commonly follows major seizures. In some temporal lobe attacks automatism may be the sole epileptic manifestation or it may occur as a prelude to a major seizure.

Affective disorders. Since the inner surface of the temporal lobe includes the limbic system, it is not surprising that disturbances of emotion may occur in temporal lobe epilepsy. These include episodes of anxiety, fear, ecstasy, depression and paranoid feelings or there may be a mixture of emotions.

A focal temporal lobe seizure may comprise but a single manifestation, or it may consist of a complicated symptomatology with much overlap. It may therefore be difficult to localise the origin of a discharge within a temporal lobe or even to lateralise it, although dysphasia suggests implication of the dominant hemisphere. The complex symptoms which have been discussed are the 'signatures' of the temporal lobe and indicate that the focal discharge originated in that part of the brain and is therefore a variety of partial epilepsy.

As in other varieties of partial epilepsy, following the focal manifestation a major seizure may develop, and in temporal lobe epilepsy this is frequently nocturnal. Not uncommonly the generalised seizure takes the form of a brief period of amnesia. If the focal manifestation of temporal lobe disorder is minimal or forgotten, temporal lobe epileptic absences may resemble petit mal but, unlike true idiopathic petit mal, there is often some postictal confusion.

A rare presentation is a *confusional state* or *apparent dementia* which may occur when there is a subclinical, cortical, electrical status epilepticus. This is completely reversible with anticonvulsant medication.

The various commoner manifestations of partial (symptomatic, focal, cortical) epilepsy are summarised in Figures 3a and b.

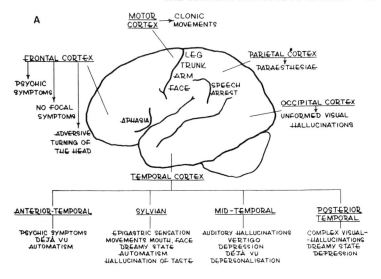

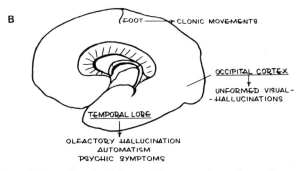

Fig. 3a and **b** Manifestations of partial (symptomatic, cortical) epilepsy.

SUMMARY

1. Generalised (usually idiopathic) **epilepsy**, due to genetic factors and less often to diffuse pathology or chemical disturbance, may result in:

    a. Absences (petit mal)
    b. Bilateral myoclonus of various types
    c. Infantile spasms
    d. Clonic seizures
    e. Tonic seizures
    f. Tonic-clonic seizures
    g. Akinetic seizures

2. Partial (symptomatic) **epilepsy** always has an underlying pathological basis.

A focal or partial → a. may remain focal
seizure: b. may spread along a gyrus
            c. may spread centrifugally
            d. may spread by cortico-thalamic pathways
              to brain stem ——→ grand mal

3. Temporal lobe epilepsy is one of the more common varieties of partial (symptomatic) epilepsy. Suspect this condition in a patient displaying one or more of these symptoms occurring in an episodic manner:

a. Epigastric sensation
b. Hallucinations of taste, smell, hearing, vision
c. Disorders of memory
d. Dreamy states
e. Disorders of affect

FURTHER READING

Andermann F 1967 Absence attacks and diffuse neuronal disease. Neurology (Minneap) 17: 205
Beatty R A 1965 The focal motor seizures as a false localising sign. Neurology (Minneap) 15: 752
Report from Boston Collaborative Drug Surveillance Program 1972. Drug induced convulsions. Lancet 2: 677
Falconer M A 1970 The pathological substrate of temporal lobe epilepsy. Guys Hosp Rep 119: 47
Halliday A M 1967 The clinical incidence of myoclonus. In: Williams E (ed) Modern trends in neurology. Butterworths, London, vol 4, p 69
Jeavons P M, Bower B D 1964 Infantile spasms. In: Clinics in developmental medicine No 15. Heinemann, London
Lance J W, Adams R D 1963 The syndrome of intention or action myoclonus as a sequel to hypoxic encephalopathy. Brain 86: 111
Lance J W 1968 Myoclonic jerks and falls: aetiology, classification and treatment. Med J Aust 1: 113
Livingstone S, Torres I, Pauli L L, Rider R V 1965 Petit mal epilepsy. J Amer Med Ass 194: 227
Penry J K, Daly D D 1976 Complex partial seizures and their treatment. Raven Press, New York
Roth M, Harper M 1962 Temporal lobe epilepsy and the phobic anxiety-depersonalisation syndrome. Comprehensive Psychiatry 3: 215
Sumi S M, Teasdall R D 1963 Focal seizures: a review of 150 cases. Neurology (Minneap) 13: 583
Williams D 1966 Temporal lobe epilepsy. Brit Med J 1: 1439

3

A note on certain varieties of epilepsy

The classification of epilepsy which forms the basis of the previous chapters is a comprehensive one and takes in all the types of epilepsy likely to be encountered in clinical practice. However, over the years other varieties of epilepsy have been named. These varieties of epilepsy are not variants of the disorder which exist over and above the types of epilepsy already described. Rather they are important clinical patterns of epilepsy which were well known before the International League's Classification of Epileptic Seizures came into use but they are not named as such in the classification. Clinicians still find it useful to refer to them so that it seems justifiable to discuss them here, indicating how they fit into the International League's classification.

REFLEX EPILEPSY

Reflex epilepsy is a term employed to indicate those varieties of epilepsy, generalised or partial, in which the seizures consistently follow some clearly defined stimulus. Use has been made of this phenomenon in electroencephalography, *overbreathing* and *photic stimulation* being employed to evoke paroxysmal E.E.G. abnormalities.

The mechanism of overbreathing in this context is uncertain but it is possible that by producing an extracellular alkalosis, overbreathing leads to a shift of Na^+ ions to inside the neurone with resulting reduction in membrane polarisation and an increased risk of neuronal discharging. Overbreathing also causes hypocapnia, which leads to intracranial vasoconstriction and decreased cerebral blood flow. These effects of overbreathing may bring out latent abnormalities of generalised or partial epilepsy. Absences (petit mal) are particularly likely to be triggered by overbreathing. Photic stimulation is effected with a stroboscope which produces high intensity flashes of light at frequencies varying from $\frac{1}{2}$ to 30 Hz close to the subject's eyes. In many normal people, stroboscope stimulation influences occipital frequencies in the electroencephalogram, so that these frequencies tend to follow the rate of flashes produced by the stroboscope. In some individuals, abnormal discharges are limited to the occipital regions, while in a few, particularly those with generalised epilepsy, widespread paroxysmal spike and wave discharges develop. It is said that Greek traders employed photic stimulation by making slaves they were about to purchase sit in front of a revolving wheel, rejecting those in whom a seizure was induced.

Photogenic epilepsy occurs clinically in a variety of circumstances which include passing from dim into bright light, driving along a tree-lined road when the sun is shining through the branches of the trees, watching a wheel revolving or a pendulum swinging and viewing television particularly from close up if the screen is disturbed by frequent flickering. A neurotic, often compulsive, response can sometimes be seen in children affected by photogenic epilepsy in that they may induce a seizure by staring at a bright light and either blinking their eyes rapidly, or waving a hand to and fro in front of their eyes. Photogenic epilepsy is a manifestation of generalised epilepsy. Another variety of reflexly-induced generalised epilepsy may occur, though rarely, after prolonged or concentrated reading (*reading epilepsy*).

Auditory stimuli may also induce reflex epilepsy. A loud noise may evoke a seizure or, as in musicogenic epilepsy, an attack may be evoked by a particular melody, the sound of a particular instrument, or even a particular peal of church bells. Musicogenic epilepsy appears to be a partial (temporal lobe) epilepsy.

Startle or touch may precipitate an epileptic attack and seizures may also be induced by *sudden movement*. This 'movement induced epilepsy' may have a familial incidence and the condition usually occurs first in childhood or adolescence. Such attacks tend to occur in response to a sudden movement like rising from a chair or beginning to run, and the seizure is characterised by a tonic spasm associated with athetoid or choreiform movements of a limb, an arm and a leg, or the entire musculature, consciousness, however, being retained. The cause is uncertain; such episodes may be a variety of generalised (often myoclonic) epilepsy, either primary or symptomatic, or they may indicate a focal lesion in the supplementary motor area of the cortex or in the basal ganglia. There is usually a satisfactory response to anticonvulsant therapy.

Occasionally *stimulation of a particular area of skin* may reflexly trigger a partial motor seizure beginning in neighbouring muscles, while stimulation of other nearby cutaneous areas may abort an induced seizure, if it has not progressed too far.

Psychological factors, particularly emotional disturbance, may evoke an epileptic attack and in some patients a particular thought may herald a seizure. (It is, however, possible that the thought may be the first symptom of a discharge from a temporal lobe). Petit mal absences and temporal lobe epilepsy are particularly emotion-sensitive. In some instances the patient may be capable of arresting the attack by consciously diverting his thoughts to something else, as for instance by concentrating intensely on counting or on a mathematical calculation. The mechanisms underlying reflex epilepsy are uncertain but it seems possible that whereas in a normal individual a given afferent stimulus produces a 'normal' response in the part of the brain to which this stimulus projects, in the potentially epileptic patient an abnormal excessive and potentially epileptogenic discharge will be evoked in this part of the brain. It is also likely that the response to an afferent stimulus depends not only on the stimulus and on the brain thus stimulated, but also on all other afferent stimuli entering the brain at the same time.

POST-TRAUMATIC EPILEPSY

It is well recognised that epilepsy may follow head injury but in considering the incidence of post-traumatic epilepsy it is necessary to subdivide such patients into (1) missile head-wounded patients and (2) closed head injury patients. The reason for this is that although reasonably precise data exist on missile wounded patients, the incidence of epilepsy as a result of closed head injuries varies widely in different published series.

Missile head injury
The overall incidence of post-traumatic epilepsy in missile head wounds is in the region of 33 per cent.

Closed (blunt; non-missile) head injury
Post-traumatic epilepsy in closed head injury patients may be classified as (1) immediate, (2) early, or (3) late.

Immediate epilepsy
This relatively rare event occurs within minutes of the trauma which is often relatively mild. There is usually only one seizure and thereafter the patient remains seizure free. This is a benign condition and the prognosis is excellent.

Early epilepsy
This may be defined as seizures occurring in the first week but not in the first minutes after the injury. It appears to be more common in the

presence of a skull fracture (particularly the depressed variety), in the presence of neurological signs of organic brain damage, and when the period of post-traumatic amnesia is prolonged. The main significance of this variety of post-traumatic epilepsy is the enhanced tendency for such patients to develop late epilepsy. There is some evidence that the exhibition of anticonvulsants for 12 to 24 months following the trauma minimises this risk.

Late epilepsy

Following closed head injuries, this entity may be defined as seizures occurring at an interval of more than one week from the time of the trauma. Although the overall risk of this condition developing is in the region of 5 per cent, the incidence varies widely according to the type of injury. Thus, early epilepsy (i.e. occurring in the first week after the trauma), or the occurrence of an intracerebral haematoma increases the risk to the 25 to 30 per cent level of probability. This rises to about 50 per cent in the presence of a depressed fracture associated with a tear in the dura together with early epilepsy, or with post-traumatic amnesia of more than 24 hours duration. In estimating the possible risks of a head injury patient developing epilepsy, the duration of post-traumatic amnesia by itself is of little importance, the three factors of most significance being the occurrence of early epilepsy, the presence of a depressed fracture, and the development of an intracerebral haematoma.

If late epilepsy does develop after a head injury, about half of the patients will have a seizure within the first two years, but in some 25 per cent the onset is delayed for more than four years from the time of the trauma. It is possible that in some instances the onset of post-traumatic epilepsy may be delayed for 20 years or more after the injury, but, in such patients, the possibility of other factors causing epilepsy should be carefully considered.

Unfortunately, unless the E.E.G. indicates a definite epileptiform focus, electroencephalography is of little value in indicating patients who may later develop post-traumatic epilepsy.

Although the seizures of post-traumatic epilepsy may be persistent and difficult to control, it is not uncommon for patients to have only a few convulsions. Indeed, in some 50 per cent of patients the course is benign and after a few years of therapy the attacks cease.

EPISODIC BEHAVIOUR DISORDERS IN CHILDREN

Behaviour disorders in children can be subdivided into two main groups, a psychogenic and a less common epileptic type, but there are also behavioural disorders resulting from a combination of psychological factors and epilepsy.

Psychogenic group

In these patients the behavioural disorders are related to genetic factors, environmental factors, parental factors or stresses associated, for example, with rivalry between siblings. Such patients (and their parents) are best treated by psychotherapeutic measures.

Epileptic group

Episodic behavioural disorders of an epileptic nature are found among children with (1) episodes of impulsive behaviour with, or without, amnesia for the episode, or with (2) paroxysms of abnormal behaviour occurring against a background of generally bad behaviour.

In this group of patients the electroencephalogram may show a non-specific excess of bilateral slow activity over the temporal lobes or posterior half of the head or paroxysmal disturbances often in the posterior temporal regions. For the disorder to be most probably epileptic it would seem that the disturbance in behaviour should occur without provocation, and that the electroencephalogram should show paroxysmal abnormalities. Improved behaviour after the intake of antiepileptic drugs is not necessarily an argument that a behaviour disorder is of epileptic origin. Antiepileptic drugs often have sedative and tranquillising properties, and any of the tranquillisers may improve behaviour disorders.

Combined psychogenic–epileptic behaviour disorders

Behavioural disorders may result from a combination of psychological and epileptic factors. The fact that they have epilepsy may set some children apart from their fellows. Psychological disturbances and behaviour disorders develop. Such children because of their difficulty in accepting normal schooling and school discipline often join fringe groups and display a tendency to antisocial activities.

It is often difficult and at times impossible to assess the percentage of aetiological contribution of these factors in the disturbances of a particular child. While a diagnostic trial of anticonvulsants is valuable in assessing epileptic factors it is obviously of considerable importance that a child should not be incorrectly labelled 'epileptic' because his behaviour improves after anticonvulsants are given.

BENIGN OR SIMPLE FEBRILE CONVULSIONS

This is a variety of generalised epilepsy which merits special consideration because of certain features, in particular the good prognosis in that such convulsions do not usually continue into the second decade of life. *The following features permit a diagnosis of benign febrile convulsions:*

1. Repeated generalised convulsions, not focal seizures, associated with, and only with, febrile illnesses.
2. A family history of convulsions associated with febrile illnesses in childhood.
3. A normal interseizure electroencephalogram and a normal neurological examination.
4. Onset usually in the first three years of life and cessation by five or six years of age.

We consider that febrile convulsions are best regarded as a variety of generalised (primary) epilepsy in which there is a constitutionally determined low seizure threshold during the first decade of life. Subsequently, the seizure threshold achieves more 'normal' levels. The great majority of children with febrile convulsions as defined above 'grow out of them'. Rarely brain damage, presumably anoxic in nature, may result from a prolonged febrile seizure. If the damaged area proves epileptogenic, partial (symptomatic) epilepsy becomes superimposed on the primary (generalised) variety, with continuance of epileptic seizures into adult life. It is therefore advisable to 'protect' children who have a tendency to febrile convulsions by administering anticonvulsant therapy.

Two approaches to treatment exist in such patients: anticonvulsants may be given at the first sign of febrile illness and discontinued when the fever settles; or anticonvulsants may be given routinely for 12 to 24 months, or longer if further convulsions occur when therapy is withdrawn. The principal disadvantage of intermittent treatment is the rapidity with which children develop a fever so that they may have a high temperature (and a febrile convulsion) before a sufficient dose of anticonvulsant can be given by the parent and absorbed by the child to provide an adequate protective drug concentration in the brain. Therefore continuous prophylaxis is preferred.

Recently it has been suggested that in some instances febrile convulsions may be due to vagally–mediated cerebral ischaemic hypoxia rather than to a direct effect of fever on the upper brain stem. Such cases may develop prolonged asystole on ocular compression.

EPILEPSY IN INFANCY AND CHILDHOOD

Special problems present themselves in the management of epilepsy in the infant and young child. The seizures tend to be atypical in the early years of life and may take the form of episodes of apnoea, limpness, tonic spasm of the limbs and trunk, unilateral tonic or clonic spasms of the limbs which may vary from one side to the other in different attacks, fixed staring, myoclonic jerks, head nodding and salaam seizures of infantile spasms. With increasing age, and increasing maturity of the nervous system, the seizures may change and finally take on the characteristics of any of the adult types of seizure.

Further, in infants and young children a single E.E.G. may prove difficult to interpret. However, serial tracings will often furnish information of value and significance.

With regard to the *aetiology* of the seizures, the age of onset is of particular significance:

In the first few months of life, causes include congenital anomalies of the brain, birth trauma, perinatal hypoxia, hypoglycaemia, and kernicterus. Hypocalcaemia should also be considered since the immature kidney has a relative inability to excrete phosphorus with resulting hyperphosphataemia and consequent hypocalcaemia. In breast fed infants, pyridoxine deficiency may occur and certain milk mixtures have been known to be deficient in vitamin B_6. Phenylketonuria may be associated with seizures, and it is in this age group that infantile spasms present.

Between six months and two years of age, benign febrile convulsions occur. In other circumstances, congenital toxoplasmosis (with chorioretinitis, hydrocephalus and mental retardation), and congenital neurosyphilis, merit consideration. One of the sequelae of encephalopathy and meningitis is epilepsy, while the presence of an organic heart lesion might suggest that the seizures are a manifestation of cerebral embolism. Occasionally, hypoglycaemia (idiopathic, due to hyperinsulinism, or to pituitary dysfunction) may present with epileptic seizures. From two years of age upwards, primary major seizures (generalised epilepsy) occur, as do focal cortical seizures (partial epilepsy) due to birth trauma, inborn errors of metabolism, arteriovenous malformations and various poisons and toxins such as lead and insecticides. From four years of age, absences may be due to hereditary generalised epilepsy (petit mal) and epilepsy in a child exposed to dogs or cats, whose blood shows an eosinophilia, may be due to toxocara canis infection.

From 5 to 15 years of age the clinical picture of deteriorating school work, change in personality and the occurrence of partial seizures or generalised seizures, usually myoclonic jerks, associated with pyramidal or extrapyramidal disturbance suggests the development of subacute sclerosing panencephalitis. (The E.E.G. often shows periodically occurring bilateral discharges consisting of solitary sharp waves).

Partial epilepsy due to brain damage at birth frequently begins in this age group.

In general, space occupying hemisphere lesions, with the exception of cerebral abscess, are not common in childhood but they do occur and the combination of partial (focal, cortical) epilepsy and papilloedema should strongly suggest the presence of a mass lesion.

SUMMARY

1. **Reflex epilepsy**—epileptic seizures which consistently follow a clearly defined stimulus such as:

   a. Overbreathing

   b. Photogenic ———┌─spontaneous
                     └─compulsive

   c. Auditory (musicogenic)

   d. Startle

   e. Specific cutaneous stimuli

   f. Psychological factors

2. **Post-traumatic epilepsy**

   a. **Missile head wounds**—about one third of patients develop epilepsy

   b. **Closed head injuries**

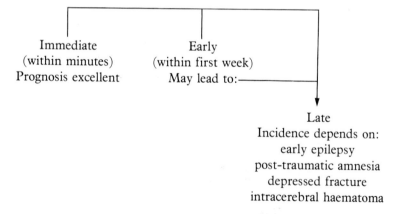

Immediate
(within minutes)
Prognosis excellent

Early
(within first week)
May lead to:————

Late
Incidence depends on:
early epilepsy
post-traumatic amnesia
depressed fracture
intracerebral haematoma

3. **Episodic behavioural disorders in children** may be:

   a. Psychogenic

   b. Epileptic

   c. Combination of (a) and (b)

4. Febrile convulsions are characterised by:

    a. Generalised convulsion associated with a pyrexial illness
    b. A family history of a similar condition
    c. Onset in first few years of life
    d. Good prognosis

5. Epilepsy in infants and children

    a. Seizures tend to be atypical in infants
    b. Serial E.E.G.s more useful than a single record
    c. Aetiological factors vary in different age groups
    d. With the exception of cerebral abscess, supratentorial tumours are uncommon in childhood but this diagnosis must be considered particularly if papilloedema is present.

FURTHER READING

Davies E 1959 Explosive or episodic behaviour disorders in children as epileptic equivalents. Med J Aust 2: 474.
Hopkins I 1972 Seizures in the first week of life. Med J Aust 2: 647
Jamieson K G 1971 A first notebook of head injury. 2nd edn. Butterworth, London
Jennett W B 1975 Epilepsy after non-missile head injuries. 2nd edn. Heinemann, London
Lennox-Buchthal M A 1973 Febrile convulsions—a reappraisal. Electroenceph. clin. Neurophysiol. Suppl. 32
Merlis J K 1974 Reflex epilepsy. In: Vinken P J, Bruyn G W (eds) Handbook of clinical neurology. North Holland Publishing Co., Amsterdam
Millichap J G 1968 Febrile convulsions. Macmillan, New York
Pallis C, Louis S 1961 Television—induced seizures. Lancet 1: 188
Stephenson J B P 1978 Two types of febrile seizures: anoxic (syncopal) and epileptic mechanisms differentiated by oculocardiac reflexes. Brit Med J 2: 726
Symonds C P 1959 Excitation and inhibition in epilepsy. Brain 82: 133
Walker A E 1962 Post traumatic epilepsy. World Neurol 3: 185

4

Conditions which may simulate epilepsy

As already indicated (p. 1) episodes suggesting impaired brain function may occur in a variety of circumstances. These include, in addition to epilepsy, disordered cerebral blood flow, disordered blood constitution, structural brain disease, the narcolepsy–cataplexy syndrome, psychoneurotic conditions and catatonic states.

DISORDERED CEREBRAL BLOOD FLOW

Syncope (fainting)
This is loss of consciousness due to acute decrease in cerebral blood flow. It is important to distinguish syncope from epilepsy and in this connection it should be remembered that a convulsion may occur if the syncopal attack is prolonged or very severe. In distinguishing syncope from epilepsy, the following signs are often helpful:

1. In syncope, pallor of the skin generally persists for some minutes after the attack.
2. The blood pressure is low and the pulse may be impalpable in a syncopal attack whereas the blood pressure is elevated or normal in epilepsy.
3. Between attacks there is usually a normal electroencephalogram in patients with syncope.
4. In syncope, the patient gives a history of 'feeling faint' ('light headed', 'cold sweat' etc.) before losing consciousness.
5. Syncope usually occurs when the patient is standing still in the upright posture.

Fainting may occur in a wide variety of conditions; some of the causes are classified in Table 5.

Breath holding attacks
These occur in children usually between 18 months and 2 years of age. An emotional disturbance, brought about by frustration or pain, leads to a bout of crying and during this a prolonged expiration is not

Table 5   Causes of syncope in different age groups

First decade of life
Simple faints related to emotion or pain
Breath holding attacks
Congenital heart disease

Adolescence
Simple faints related to emotion or pain
Hysterical overbreathing
Standing erect on a hot day
Complicated migraine

Adult life

Cardiovascular conditions
Simple faints in relation to emotion or pain
Paroxysmal tachycardia
Heart block (Stokes-Adams attacks)
Valvular heart disease (e.g. aortic stenosis)
Carotid sinus syncope
Vertebro-basilar insufficiency

Respiratory conditions
Cough syndrome
Primary pulmonary hypertension

Postural hypotension
Idiopathic
Prolonged standing
Pregnancy
Haemorrhage
Hypotensive drugs
Micturition syncope

followed by inspiration. The child becomes unconscious and may twitch or even convulse. Within a few seconds, however, consciousness is regained and the child is again well. The mechanism is probably similar to that of the fainting lark of schoolboys in which hyperventilation leads to cerebral vaso-constriction and holding the breath in expiration to a fall in blood pressure, the combined effect resulting in cerebral anoxia. In the fainting lark, however, there may be in addition decreased venous return to the heart due to increased intrathoracic pressure.

Overbreathing episodes
Hysterical overbreathing which may occur in schoolgirls, even in epidemic proportion, may result in dizziness, fainting and symptoms of tetany.

Carotid sinus syncope

This usually affects middle aged males and is characterised by vertigo or syncope immediately following movements of, or pressure on, the neck. The diagnosis may be made by reproducing the patient's symptoms by gentle massage over the carotid sinus on one or other side (the sinus is usually located in relation to the arterial pulse at the upper border of the thyroid cartilage). In the presence of a hypersensitive carotid sinus there is abrupt slowing of the heart, a fall in blood pressure, or both. Carotid sinus syncope may occur in relation to atherosclerotic changes in the carotid artery, or in inflammatory lesions or tumours of the neck.

Pressure over one carotid artery may produce symptoms of cerebral ischaemia if the other carotid artery is not fully patent, and attacks of impaired consciousness (typically 'drop attacks') may occur on movement of the neck in patients with vertebro-basilar occlusive disease particularly when this condition is associated with cervical spondylosis.

Complicated migraine

In one variant of this condition, loss of consciousness is referable to vasomotor changes in the basilar artery producing brain stem ischaemia. More rarely, cerebral ischaemia from migrainous vaso-spasm may activate an epileptic seizure in a potentially epileptic brain.

Cardiac conditions

In infants, syncopal attacks may indicate the presence of congenital heart disease, and in older children loss of consciousness after exertion is more likely to be due to a cardiac abnormality than epilepsy. In a patient experiencing *syncopal attacks in relation to exertion* one of the following conditions may be responsible:

1. Congenital heart disease.
2. Aortic or mitral stenosis.
3. Myocardial failure.
4. Primary pulmonary hypertension.

Other cardiac lesions which may be associated with episodes of fainting include myocardial infarction, paroxysmal tachycardia and heart block.

Coughing

Syncopal attacks associated with coughing were first described by Charcot. This condition is now generally referred to as cough syndrome or cough syncope. Middle aged, plethoric, thick-set males, addicted to smoking and alcohol, are generally affected. A severe bout of coughing without taking a breath between coughs results in increased intrathoracic pressure, decreased cardiac filling pressure and decreased cardiac output. It seems probable that in many cases the cerebral circulation is also embarrassed by stenotic changes particularly in the vertebro-basilar system. Thus cough syndrome results from transient impairment of cardiac output in a patient whose cerebral blood flow is already compromised. In other instances, cough syndrome may be associated with a hypersensitive carotid sinus; in a few a slight cough may be the initial symptom of an epileptic discharge ('laryngeal epilepsy'—a form of reflex epilepsy); in others, cerebral ischaemia resulting from coughing may activate a latent epileptogenic focus and even suggest the presence of a hitherto 'silent' cerebral tumour.

Blood loss
All normal humans will faint if sufficient blood volume is lost, for example, by haemorrhage. Loss of effective blood volume is also the cause of syncope after prolonged standing and in syncope associated with the use of some hypotensive drugs, in that in effect the individual 'bleeds into the veins of the lower part of his body' when blood pools in these vessels. *Micturition syncope*, in which middle aged or elderly males lose consciousness on passing urine, usually after getting out of bed at night for this purpose, probably has a similar mechanism. Blood is pooled in the dilated peripheral circulation, and then venous return to the heart falls abruptly when intra-abdominal pressure falls once the bladder is emptied. Similarly, conditions of vasodilatation (e.g. leaving a warm bed or hot bath), particularly when associated with a moderate valsalva manoeuvre, resulting in a rise of intrathoracic pressure (e.g. straining at stool), may cause a syncopal attack in either sex.

DISORDERED BLOOD CONSTITUTION

Severe anaemia (with the exception of that produced by acute haemorrhage) is relatively uncommon nowadays. A much more common cause in this category is *overdosage* with sedative drugs. This, of course, tends to produce a period of prolonged stupor or coma rather than episodes of unconsciousness, unless repeated overdoses are taken. In such patients it is always advisable to have the serum levels of barbiturate, bromide and other commonly used psychotrophic drugs estimated and the presence of these drugs and their metabolites in urine checked. Withdrawal of barbiturates in patients who have become dependent and are overdosing not uncommonly results in either a single or a series of major convulsive seizures.

Delirium tremens and deliria due to other causes may also be associated with major seizures.

Hypoglycaemia
This merits consideration in patients who present with any of the following:

1. Disturbance of consciousness.
2. Voracious appetite.
3. Transient neurological defects.
4. Paroxysmal disorders of behaviour.
5. Symptoms of alcoholism but who deny taking alcohol.
6. Epileptic seizures (focal or generalised).

Hypoglycaemia may be due to physiological (e.g. after gastric resection), organic (e.g. islet cell adenoma of pancreas) or miscellaneous causes (e.g. overdosage with insulin, inanition). A blood sugar of under 50 mg/100 ml and prompt relief when glucose (20 ml, 50 per cent) is administered intravenously strongly favour this diagnosis.

Parathyroid insufficiency
This may present to the neurologist with fits and papilloedema. There is, in addition, usually evidence of tetany, latent or overt. In some patients, there may be calcification in the basal ganglia. Since the fits and papilloedema may be controlled and abolished by the administration of parathormone or calciferol it seems possible that hypocalcaemia and excessive cerebral hydration are responsible for these symptoms. This condition, like seizures associated with hypoglycaemia, can be regarded as a form of epilepsy resulting from extracranial causes.

STRUCTURAL BRAIN DISEASE

Organic lesions producing impaired consciousness rather than epileptic seizures occur most frequently in relation to the brain stem, and particularly with lesions near the third and fourth ventricles. Epilepsy is a common symptom of tumours of the hemispheres but is rare in tumours of the brain stem; when it does occur in brain stem lesions it is generally secondary to increased intracranial pressure, and disturbance of function of the reticular formation. Tumours of the upper brain stem or thalamus have been reported to produce disorders of consciousness which may be continuous or intermittent, and 'drop attacks' (sudden loss of postural tone) may occur in posterior fossa lesions—basilar artery insufficiency, aneurysm or tumour.

Paroxysmal positional vertigo is occasionally due to lesions in the region of the fourth ventricle; very much more often it is related to pathology in the utricle of one inner ear related to trauma, vestibular neuronitis or occurring for no detectable reason. The transient but severe rotational vertigo, without loss of consciousness, which occurs when the head is placed in a particular position (e.g. getting into or out of bed: rolling over in bed) may be confused with brief attacks of epilepsy. With the vertigo there is a paroxysm of rotational nystagmus with the quick phase towards the affected ear, and the condition can be provoked by moving the head backwards from the erect to the supine position and turning the head so that the affected ear faces down.

NARCOLEPSY—CATAPLEXY SYNDROME

Although narcolepsy is not a common condition the correct diagnosis is important since, while embarrassing or even dangerous to the patient, narcolepsy itself generally responds to therapy. In its fully developed form, the syndrome comprises four separate conditions— narcolepsy, cataplexy, sleep paralysis and hypnagogic hallucinations. Narcolepsy and cataplexy are frequently associated but any of these conditions may occur independently and the link between them probably lies in some disturbance of the reticular formation or a functionally related part of the upper brain stem. The majority of these patients shows no evidence of organic neurological disease and the electroencephalogram generally furnishes records similar to light sleep occurring intermittently during the recording. Some cases of narcolepsy are related to head injury or encephalitis.

Narcolepsy

This affects both sexes (males being slightly more often affected than females), and generally starts by the third decade of life. It is characterised by episodes of irresistible sleep which may last for minutes to an hour or two. The attacks often occur in situations in which normal people often feel sleepy (e.g. after meals or during a monotonous meeting) but also at inappropriate times (e.g. when driving a car).

Cataplexy

This comprises attacks of abrupt loss of postural tone in which the patient experiences a feeling of weakness and falls to the ground but remains fully conscious. These episodes are stimulated by emotion such as laughter, anger or excitement.

Sleep paralysis
In these episodes, which occur predominantly in males, the patient experiences attacks of complete loss of muscle power usually as he wakens from sleep but sometimes just before he falls asleep. Although conscious he remains unable to move a limb for a minute or two or unless he is relieved by being touched.

Hypnagogic hallucinations
These are vivid auditory or visual hallucinations which generally occur just as the patient is going to sleep.

PSYCHIATRIC CONDITIONS

Epilepsy may be associated with a variety of psychiatric conditions which will be discussed in a later section of the book; we are here concerned with differentiating between epilepsy and hysterical seizures. When considering this topic the words of Jean-Martin Charcot might well be recalled. 'I should like, since the opportunity is at hand, to remind you of the great difference there is in the clinical form as well as in the substratum of an epileptic attack when compared to an attack of hysteroepilepsy'. Charcot continued, 'My respect for tradition has made me use the term hysteroepilepsy in the past, but I must confess it bothers me because it is absurd.'

Charcot, however, encountered patients in whom it was difficult to distinguish between epilepsy and hysterical seizures, and this difficulty can be appreciated when it is recalled that in the Salpetriere at that time epileptics and hysterics were housed in the same department. It would thus be natural for the hysterics to mimic the epileptic seizures which they had witnessed. Even with modern techniques it is sometimes difficult to determine when hysterical fits (pseudoseizures) end and epilepsy begins. The correct diagnosis may emerge if consideration is given to the various factors indicated in Table 6.

The question as to whether a seizure is epileptic or hysterical in nature is, however, often an over-simplification. One or other of the following relationships may occur.

1. The patient may be suffering from epilepsy, or the seizure may be hysterical in nature (a 'pseudoseizure').
2. Epilepsy and an hysterical reaction may co-exist as two separate aetiologically unrelated entities in the one individual.
3. Epilepsy may result in an hysterical reaction. This would seem to be particularly true of temporal lobe epilepsy.
4. An hysterical disturbance may activate an epileptic seizure—an affective reflex epilepsy.

Catatonic states may be due to frontal lobe lesions—the so-called akinetic mutism, or to schizophrenia. Such states are rare but can be confused with the equally rare cortical epileptic status or absence status in adults.

Table 6 Differential diagnosis between epilepsy and hysterical seizures (pseudoseizures)

	Epilepsy	Hysterical seizure
Occurrence of the seizure	Alone or in company: at night (when asleep) or during the day	Usually in relation to an emotional upset and usually in company
The seizure	Usually conforms to one of the classical types. Patient may bite tongue or otherwise injure himself	Often bizarre Tongue rarely bitten
Complexion during seizure	Cyanosis or pallor	Often no change
Incontinence during seizure	Common	Very rare
Corneal reflexes during seizure	Absent	Present
Plantar responses during seizure	Often extensor	Flexor
E.E.G.	Abnormal potentials almost always occur during an attack and usually occur between attacks	Tracing may be normal or non-specifically abnormal but not paroxysmal: further changes do not occur during attacks

SUMMARY

Conditions which may simulate epilepsy include:

1. Disordered cerebral blood flow ⟶ loss of consciousness

= Syncope

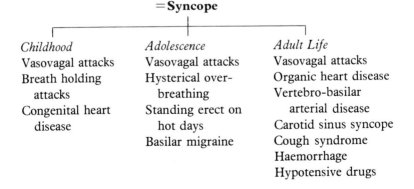

Childhood	*Adolescence*	*Adult Life*
Vasovagal attacks	Vasovagal attacks	Vasovagal attacks
Breath holding attacks	Hysterical over-breathing	Organic heart disease
Congenital heart disease	Standing erect on hot days	Vertebro-basilar arterial disease
	Basilar migraine	Carotid sinus syncope
		Cough syndrome
		Haemorrhage
		Hypotensive drugs

2. Disordered blood constitution

  a. Anaemia
  b. Sedative Drugs
  c. Hypoglycaemia
    (i) functional
    (ii) islet cell adenoma ⎤ may produce secondary
    (iii) inanition   ⎥ extracranial epilepsy
    (iv) insulin overdose ⎦
  d. Hypoparathyroidism

3. Structural brain disease

Encephalopathy ⎤
Cysts   ⎥ In relation to brain stem and third
Tumours   ⎦ ventricle

Paroxysmal positional vertigo ⎯⎤⎯ Utricle
                                     ⎦⎯ Fourth ventricle region

4. Narcolepsy—cataplexy syndrome

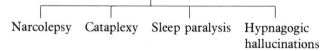

Narcolepsy   Cataplexy   Sleep paralysis   Hypnagogic
                                             hallucinations

5. Psychiatric conditions

Hysterical 'pseudoseizures': Catatonic states.

FURTHER READING

Allsop J L 1973 Carotid Sinus Syncope. Proc Aust Assoc Neurol 10: 7
Bickerstaff E R 1961 Impairment of consciousness in migraine. Lancet 2: 1057
Bickerstaff E R 1961 Basilar artery migraine. Lancet 1: 15
Bowling G, Richards N G 1961 Narcolepsy. Cleveland Clin Quart 28: 38
Eadie M J 1967 Paroxysmal positional giddiness. Med J Aust 1: 1169
Eadie M J 1968 Some aspects of episodic giddiness. Med J Aust 2: 453
Hutchinson E C, Stock J P P 1960 The carotid sinus syndrome. Lancet 2: 445
Liske E, Forster F M 1964 Pseudoseizures; a problem in the diagnosis and
   management of epileptic patients. Neurology (Minneap) 14: 41
Moss P D, McEvedy C P 1966 An epidemic of overbreathing among schoolgirls.
   Brit Med J 2: 1295
Sharpey-Schafer E P 1953 The mechanism of syncope after coughing. Brit Med J 2: 860
Sharpey-Schafer E P 1956 Syncope. Brit Med J 1: 506
Sutherland J M, Bowman D A, Tyrer J H 1965 Cough Syncope. Med J Aust 1: 39
Sutherland J M, Tyrer J H, Eadie M J 1966 Hypoglycaemia resulting from insulin
   secreting tumours of the pancreas. Proc Aust Assoc Neurol 4: 69
Tyrer J H 1957 The differentiation of hysteria from organic neurological disease.
   Med J Aust 1: 566
Willison R G, Whitty C W M 1957 Parathyroid deficiency presenting as epilepsy
   Brit Med J 1: 802

5

Investigations in epilepsy

When a patient presents with a story suggestive of epilepsy, the clinician should follow the usual routine of history taking, clinical examination, differential diagnosis, ancillary investigations and diagnosis.

HISTORY

A full history should be taken with particular reference to subjective experiences preceding the seizure and to postictal phenomena such as confusion, headache, sleepiness. It may be necessary to ask direct questions regarding, for example, epigastric sensations, hallucinations or déjà vu experiences. Patients readily omit to mention such symptoms either because they feel that these experiences are not relevant, or because they believe that abnormal experiences of vision or hearing may incline the doctor to a psychiatric diagnosis. Information should also be sought about precipitating factors, the time when attacks usually occur, and the occurrence of urinary incontinence, tongue biting or other injuries sustained during the seizures. It is also of great importance to obtain an eye-witness account of events which occurred during attacks.

It will be appreciated that a history of cortical events whether motor, sensory or psychic, preceding a generalised seizure indicates the high probability of a partial (symptomatic) epilepsy of cortical origin, whereas associated symptoms of sleepiness, sweating, hunger and confusion may suggest an extracranial aetiology, such as hypoglycaemia. On the other hand, it will be recalled that the absence of a history of an aura does not exclude the possibility that the initial epileptic discharge may have originated from cortical neurones.

In patients with epilepsy, the previous history and family history may contain highly relevant information. For example, a history of a difficult or traumatic birth or of a significant head injury later in life may suggest a traumatic basis for the epilepsy. Similarly, a history of meningitis, of encephalitis or of syphilis may be of aetiological importance while, in older age groups, a history of symptoms referable to cerebrovascular or cardiovascular disease may suggest that epilepsy has a basis in cerebral ischaemia. However, a history of head injury in the past does not render the patient immune to the later development of a cerebral tumour. Further, in some instances head trauma leads to the development of a porencephalic cyst or extremely rarely to a meningioma which may be amenable to surgery. Thus, careful assessment is necessary before a diagnosis of post-traumatic epilepsy due to a cortical cicatrix is made. On the other hand, a family history of epilepsy would tend to suggest a primary (genetic) variety, particularly if the seizure pattern is consistent with a variety of generalised epilepsy.

EXAMINATION

In a few instances a probable aetiological diagnosis can be made as the patient walks into the consulting room, or from the end of the patient's bed. This can be achieved, for example, in patients suffering from:

1. Tuberose sclerosis (Figs. 4a and b).
2. Neurofibromatosis (Fig. 5).
3. Encephalo-facial angiomatosis i.e. the Sturge-Weber syndrome (Figs. 6a and b).
4. Hemifacial atrophy (Figs. 7a and b).

In other patients, the underlying pathology may be suggested by findings on neurological examination. Aside from obvious evidence of intracranial disease such as papilloedema or signs of focal cerebral disorder, significance would attach to the presence of Argyll-Robertson pupils, a cephalic bruit in a patient older than 10 years of age, or evidence of occlusive cerebrovascular disease.

It must be emphasised, however, that the occurrence of epilepsy for the first time in middle life should arouse suspicion of a cerebral tumour. This possibility should not be discounted because there are no abnormal physical signs on neurological examination, because there is a previous history of head injury, because there is evidence of cerebrovascular occlusive disease or because the seizures have been controlled by anticonvulsant therapy. In all such patients, following a full physical and neurological examination, minimal ancillary investigations should include X-rays of skull, X-rays of chest, electroencephalography and computerised tomographic (C.T.) scanning of the head or radio-isotopic (gamma) brain scanning.

ELECTROENCEPHALOGRAPHY

The E.E.G. is of considerable value in assessing the type of epilepsy and of some value in determining its aetiology. As with any investigation it must be only one factor in the overall clinical assessment. A normal E.E.G. does not exclude a diagnosis of epilepsy when there is a clear description of an epileptic event from an observer (Fig. 8). A report of slow waves in a temporal region consistent with epileptogenic activity does not mean the patient is necessarily suffering from temporal lobe epilepsy (Fig. 9).

The E.E.G. by and large records only potentials over the surface of the cerebral convexities. These potentials, however, reflect to a considerable extent activity in the upper brain stem and thalamus. Thus epileptogenic activity arising in areas of cortex medially and inferiorly in the hemispheres is usually not readily detected in the E.E.G. unless this activity projects into, and activates, the meso-diencephalic reticular formation. Because of this, special techniques are used when indicated, e.g. sphenoidal recordings are made with needle electrodes inserted under the sphenoidal ridges to detect epileptogenic activity in the inferomedial surface of the temporal lobe and depth recordings are effected by inserting a bundle of electrodes through a burr hole in the skull.

The E.E.G. is recordable from the time of birth. (Foetal brain potentials are detectable but at the moment there is little clinical application of such recording). With maturation of the brain there is a progressive shift of dominant frequency range from slow, theta activity (4 to 7 Hz) to the alpha rhythm (8 to 13 Hz in occipital regions) and fast (beta) activity, (14 to 30 Hz) present in adult life (Figs. 10 and 11). As with other physiological measurements there is a range of normal variation in the E.E.G. at any age. Persistence of slow activity, normal for age group, into an older age group, occurs and is sometimes known as a 'maturational' defect.

A degree of cooperation and relaxation is necessary from the patient to obtain an awake recording. Many young children and particularly those who are hyperkinetic (as are some children with epilepsy) are incapable of this and require sedation to produce sleep (Fig. 15). There is a substantial variation from child to child in the amount of sedation required so that by the time sufficient sedation has been given (perhaps in repeated doses) and becomes effective a recording may have occupied several hours. Although barbiturates may be undesirable from other points of view, a short-acting barbiturate (e.g. quinalbarbitone) has a particular advantage from the E.E.G. point of view. Such a drug causes cortical fast rhythm to be superimposed on the sleeping E.E.G., and if there is an area of non-functioning cortex such induced fast rhythm may be absent locally.

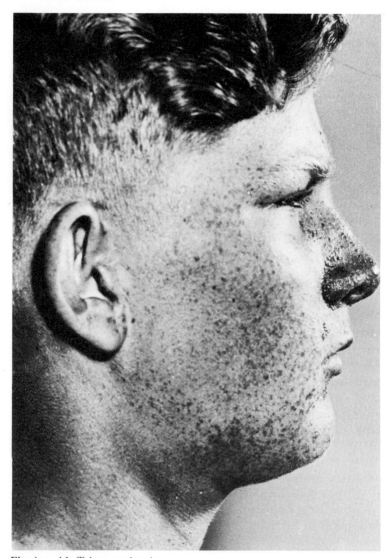

Fig. 4a and **b** Tuberose sclerosis.

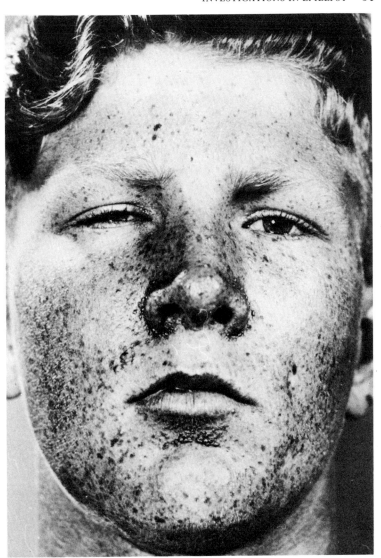

Fig. 4b

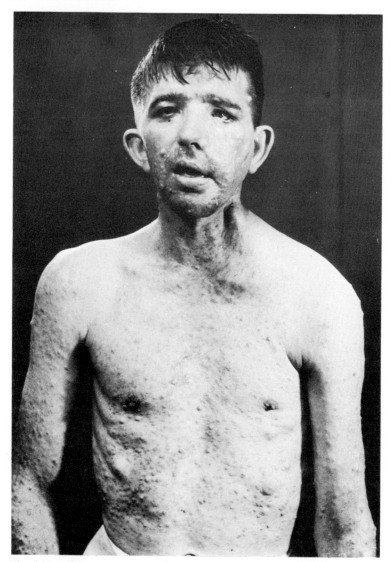

Fig. 5 Neurofibromatosis.

As sleep becomes deeper, increasingly slow activity develops over the cerebral surface until with deep sleep there is diffuse delta (1 to 3 Hz) activity (Figs. 14 and 15). While sleep tends to activate temporal lobe epileptogenic activity, the generalised slow activity may obscure the focal slow activity due to a destructive lesion.

Actual seizures are recorded infrequently. Brain epileptogenic electrical activity is episodic, but may be present, however, much of the time in between clinical seizures. The usefulness of the E.E.G. in epilepsy is largely dependent on these interseizure abnormalities. To increase the likelihood of these being detected, various activation techniques are used, e.g., hyperventilation, photic stimulation, sleep recordings with barbiturates, excitation with intravenous pentylenetetrazole (Metrazol).

Overall then, the E.E.G. provides information on the electrical behaviour of some parts of the brain at the time of the recording. It is thus a limited physiological or pathophysiological test rather than a diagnostic one.

Further problems may arise because E.E.G. reporting is to an extent subjective (reports on the same tracing varying on occasion from one reporter to another) and because the referring physician may infer more from a report than the reporter intends.

Ideally all physicians using E.E.G.s should report their own tracings as this makes easier the assessment of how much significance to give a particular tracing in the overall assessment of a patient. In practice most E.E.G.s are interpreted by E.E.G. reporters. Reports are usually made in two parts— a description (of wave form, frequencies and their locations) and the interpretation or opinion. This will almost certainly be more useful and informative if an adequate history has been provided. An adequate history is necessary also if the most useful activation techniques are to be decided on.

Sometimes patients are incorrectly diagnosed as 'epileptic' on the basis of an ill-defined history of a turn and an E.E.G. report 'consistent with epilepsy' while others are incorrectly regarded as normal when there is a similar history and a normal E.E.G. report. The E.E.G. at times can be quite misleading.

Provided the usefulness and limitations of the E.E.G. are recognised, it is the most useful test in the preliminary investigation of epilepsy and should be carried out on all patients. Serial E.E.G.s and special techniques are indicated in particular situations.

E.E.G. patterns

Epilepsy arising from the upper brain stem (that is, generalised epilepsy), particularly when primary (that is, hereditary), is typically

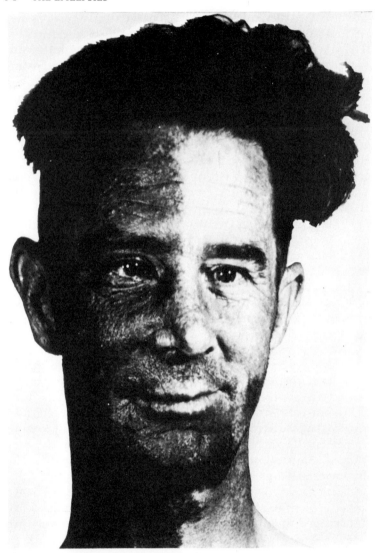

Fig. 6a and **b** Encephalo-facial angiomatosis.

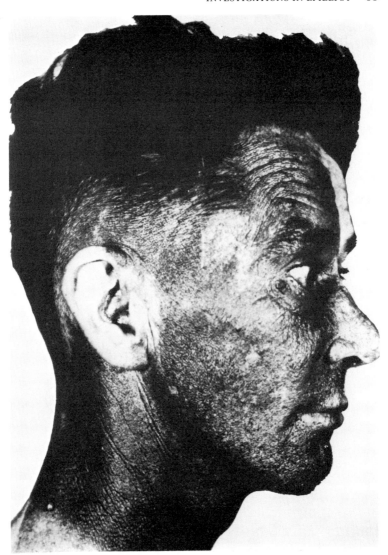

Fig. 6b

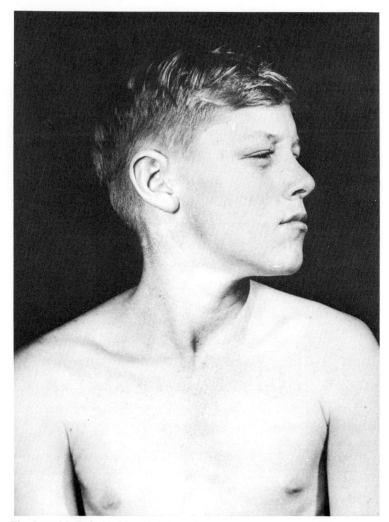

Fig. 7a and **b** Left sided hemifacial atrophy.

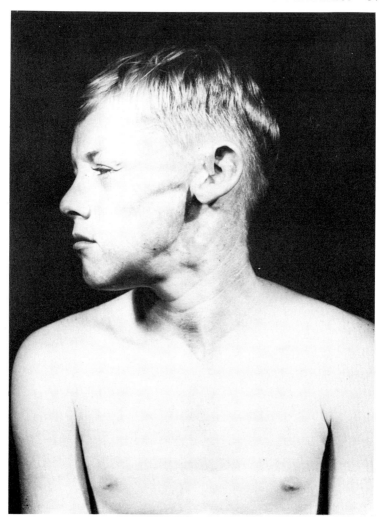

Fig. 7b

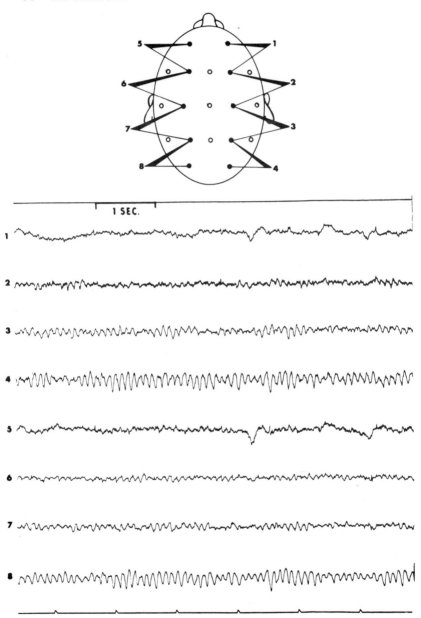

Fig. 8 Normal E.E.G. The patient had epilepsy.

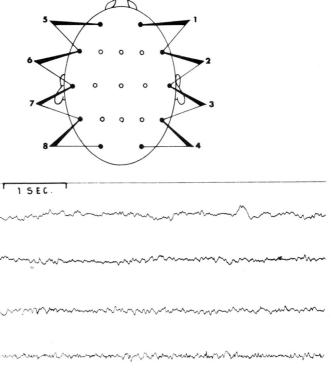

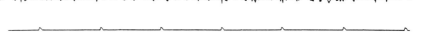

Fig. 9 Slow wave abnormality left temporal region consistent with epilepsy. The patient had migraine, not epilepsy.

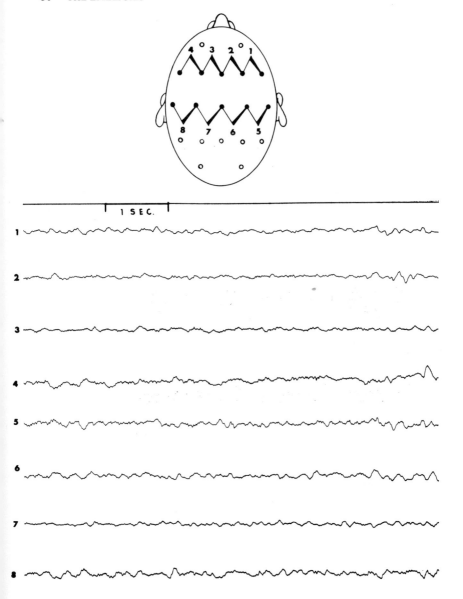

Fig. 10 Normal child aged 4; diffuse theta activity.

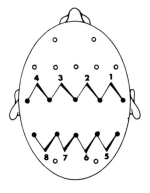

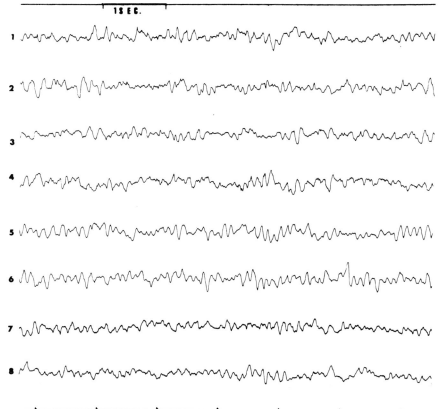

Fig. 11 Normal child aged 10; alpha rhythm and some diffuse theta activity.

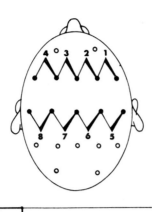

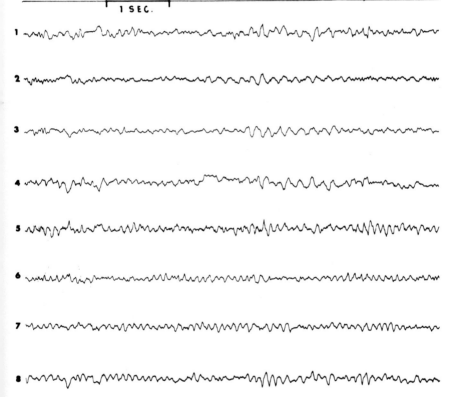

Fig. 12 Excess bilateral frontal and anterior temporal theta activity in a 22 year old psychopath.

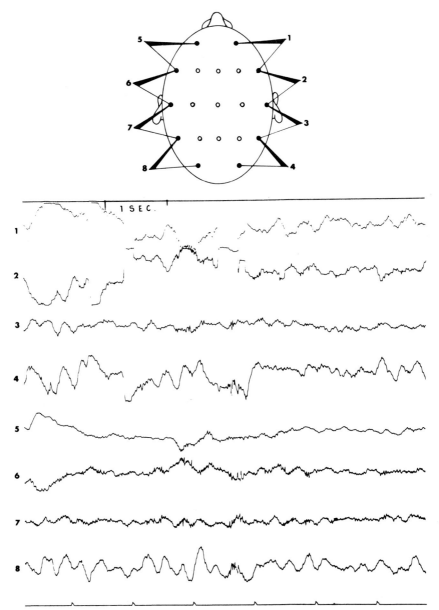

Fig. 13 Artefact; muscle (fine spikes) and frontal electrode movement. A restless baby.

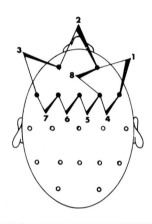

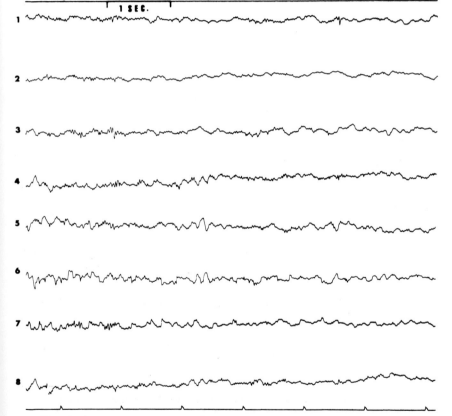

Fig. 14 Light sleep; bilateral theta activity and fast activity due to barbiturate. Child aged 6.

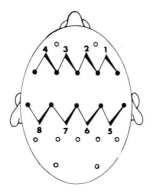

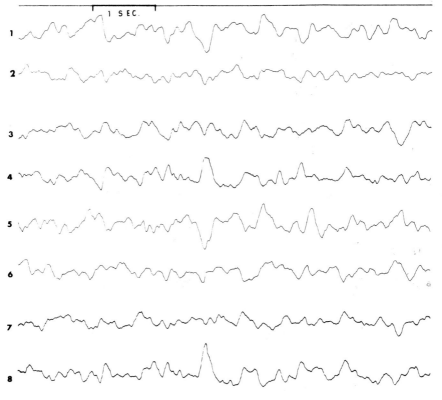

Fig. 15 Deep sleep; diffuse theta and delta activity. Child age 6.

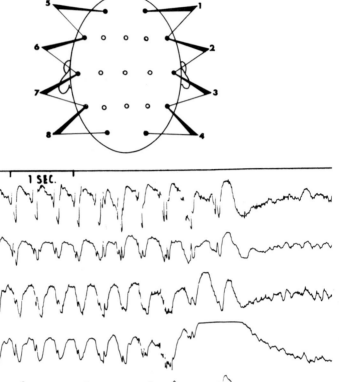

Fig. 16 Generalised epilepsy, petit mal absence. Generalised mainly regular spike and slow wave complexes at 3 Hz reverting to normal rhythms. Child aged 10; no clinical attacks for one year.

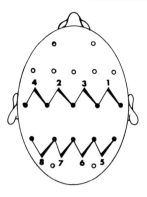

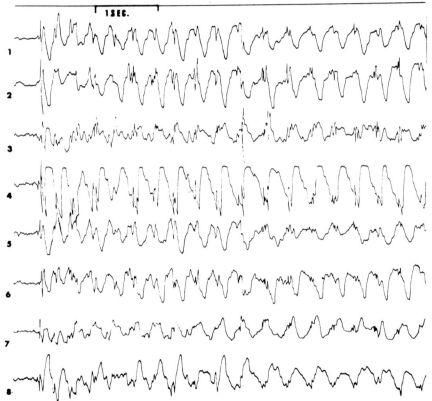

Fig. 17 Generalised epilepsy, myoclonic attacks. Generalised polyspike and slow wave complexes at varying frequencies. Child aged 11; frequent clinical attacks uncontrolled by medication.

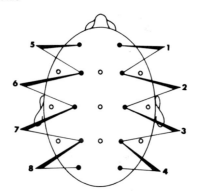

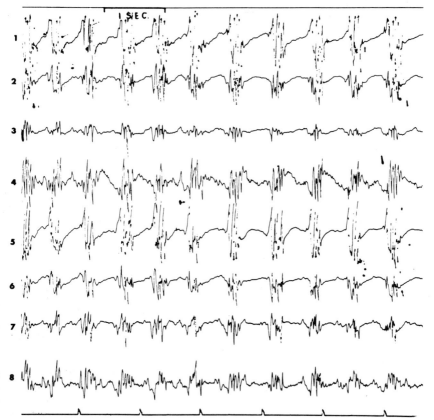

Fig. 18 Generalised epilepsy, major seizure (grand mal), clonic phase. Generalised bursts of spikes. Man aged 50.

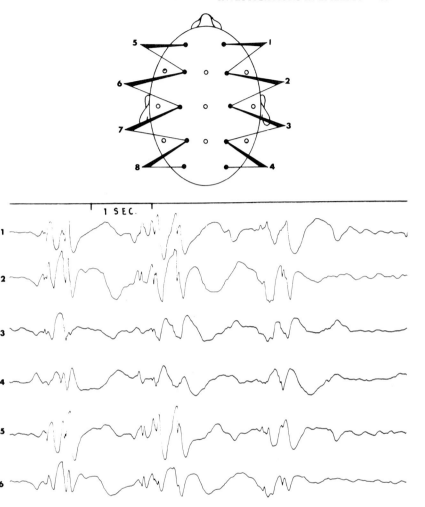

Fig. 19 Generalised epilepsy, hypsarrhythmia, sleep record. Bursts of sharp waves and slow waves, alternating with periods of low voltage activity. Child aged 2, microcephalic and mentally retarded, suffered from infantile spasms from 6 months of age.

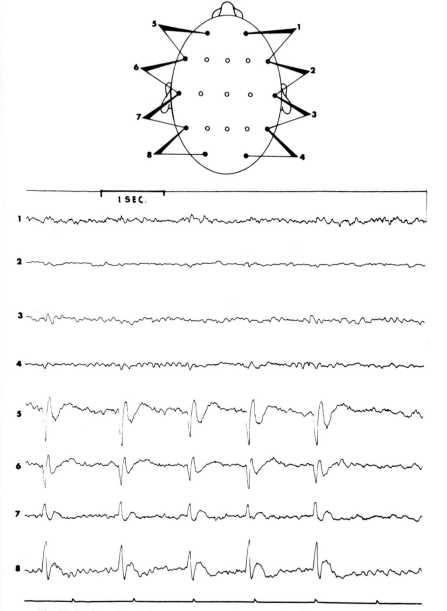

Fig. 20 Partial epilepsy (focal cortical). Phase reversals between spikes at the left mid-temporal electrode. Child aged 10 with temporal lobe epilepsy probably due to birth trauma.

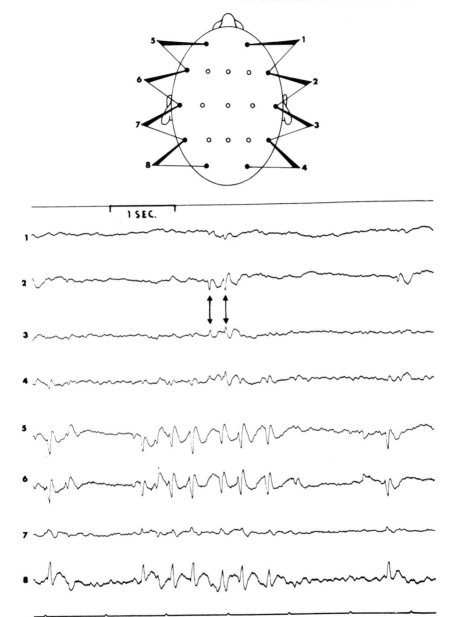

Fig. 21 Partial epilepsy (focal cortical). Male aged 16 with long standing grand mal as well as left temporal lobe seizures. A right sided 'mirror' discharge is present (arrows).

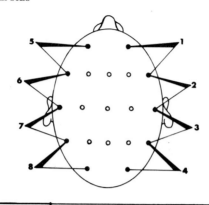

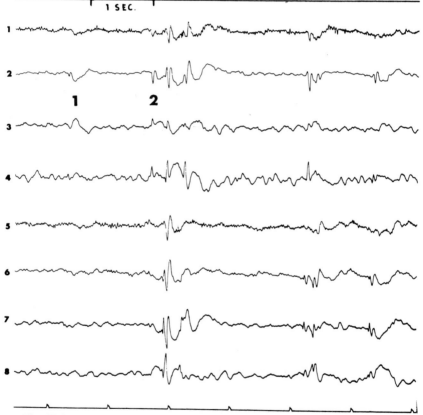

Fig. 22 Partial epilepsy. Epileptic focus right mid-temporal region. The second focal discharge (2) is rapidly followed by a bilateral spike and wave discharge. Woman aged 42; cause of epilepsy not determined.

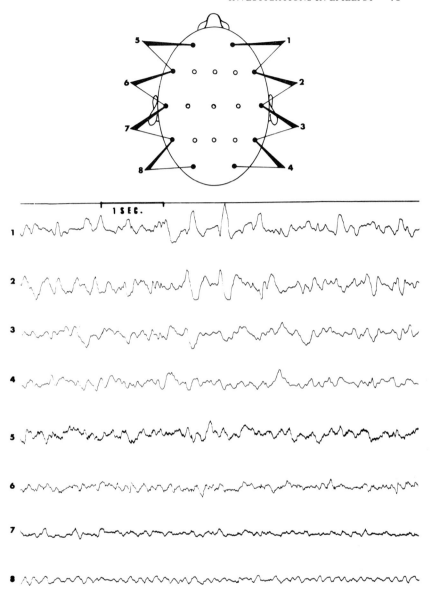

Fig. 23 Right fronto-temporal neoplasm. Delta and theta activity and sharp waves of partial (symptomatic cortical) epilepsy at the right anterior temporal electrode. Male aged 45 with secondary melanoma.

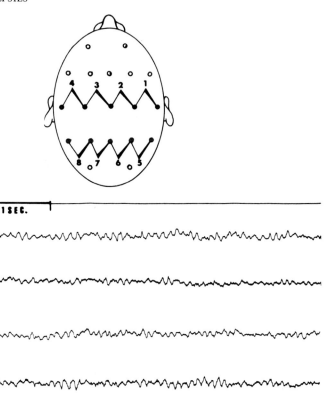

Fig. 24 Normal E.E.G. Female aged 48 with deep right parietal neoplasm and grand mal seizures.

associated with diffuse bilaterally synchronous 3 Hz spike and wave discharges over the cortex with voltage maxima anteriorly (Fig. 16) whereas partial (focal cortical) epilepsy is associated with discharges over the affected area (Fig. 20). Such localised activity may spread by interhemisphere connections to produce a 'mirror' discharge in the opposite hemisphere (Fig. 21). From assessment of type and location of these discharges considerable information is obtained on type and area of origin of some seizures.

The E.E.G. is of less value in assessing aetiology. Any pathological process which destroys or temporarily impairs function of neurones tends to produce slow activity. Thus an intracerebral haemorrhage, a contusion due to head injury, an abscess or expansion of a rapidly growing glioma may all produce similar E.E.G. patterns (Fig. 23). Serial E.E.G.s can help determine progression or regression of the process and thus help determine its aetiology. A slowly growing surface meningioma or rapidly growing deep glioma may produce no E.E.G. abnormality even though it is of substantial size (Fig. 24). Dead neurones produce no electrical activity whereas those being destroyed or whose function is being impaired produce slow activity. This can lead to incorrect localisation of the centre of a neoplasm, since the main abnormality may be at the margin of the tumour. Projected activity to the cortex of the opposite frontal lobe from an expanding lesion deep in the hemisphere may even lead to incorrect lateralisation, while a mass lesion in the cerebral hemispheres producing distortion of the upper brain stem may cause projected bilateral frontal 'rhythm at a distance' from the primary pathology.

Generalised E.E.G. disturbances (mostly slow activity) result from a wide variety of disturbances of brain stem function. These include such widely divergent conditions as brain stem contusion, expanding lesions in the region of the third ventricle, brain stem displacement whether due to supratentorial or subtentorial lesions, vascular insufficiency, biochemical disturbances as in hepatic or renal failure, hypoxia or hypoglycaemia, narcolepsy, sedative drugs and even ordinary marked drowsiness.

The E.E.G. overall is safe and painless and is a very useful test provided its limitations are well understood.

RADIOGRAPHY

X-rays of skull
Plain X-rays of the skull provide information of diagnostic value in only a relatively small proportion of patients. However, radiographs of the skull may furnish evidence of the following conditions.

Increased intracranial pressure

Children. This may be demonstrated by separation of sutures or changes in the dorsum sellae (late).

Adults. Changes in the dorsum sellae suggest increased intracranial pressure while displacement of a calcified pineal may lateralise a mass lesion.

(Note: the presence of increased convolutional markings, unless very well developed, is by itself of doubtful significance.)

Intracranial calcification

Physiological. Intracranial calcification may be physiological, e.g., pineal; choroid plexus.

Pathological. The calcification may have a pathological significance

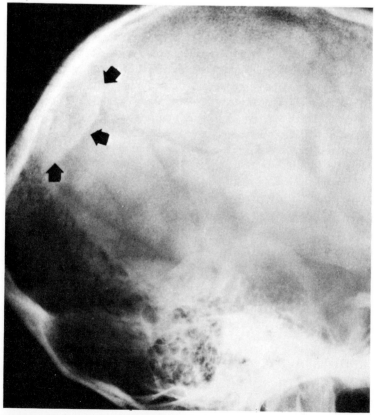

Fig. 25a Plain X-ray of skull showing hyperostosis in posterior parietal-parasaggital region, suggesting the presence of underlying meningioma.

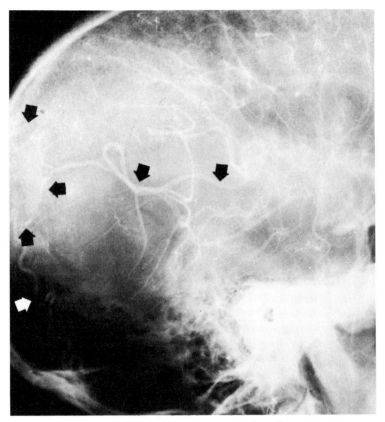

Fig. 25b Angiogram showing arterial supply to meningioma from enlarged branches (middle meningeal and occipital) of the external carotid artery.

e.g., arteriovenous malformation; a calcified cyst—dermoid or parasitic; meningioma (Fig. 25); craniopharyngioma.

Local erosion
There are several conditions in which local erosion may occur e.g., the internal auditory meatus in an acoustic neuroma, the sella turcica in pituitary adenoma or the vault in meningioma or myeloma.

Hyperostosis
This may be no pathological significance or may occur in relation to a meningioma or a generalised disorder such as Paget's disease of bone.

X-rays of chest
In the present context, X-rays of the chest are usually taken to exclude a primary carcinoma of lung which may have metastasised to the brain.

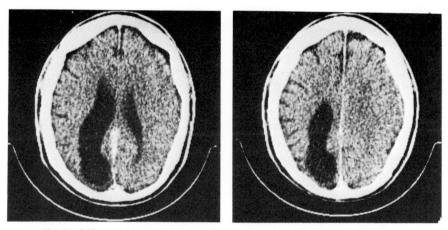

Fig. 26 C.T. scan showing dilatation of the body and occipital horn of the left lateral ventricle with some left sided cerebral cortical atrophy in a patient who developed right sided epileptic seizures following encephalitis.

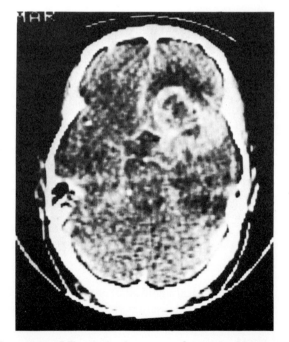

Fig. 27 Post-contrast C.T. scan showing an area of contrast enhancement due to a glioblastoma in the right frontal and temporal regions, with an area of decreased radiological density (cerebral oedema) more anteriorly. The patient had epilepsy.

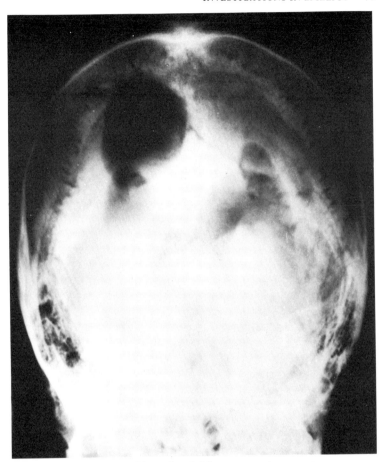

Fig. 28 Air encephalogram: The patient is lying prone to demonstrate a porencephalic cyst in relation to the left occipital horn. There is a fracture line in the parieto-occipital region.

The presence of other pulmonary pathologies, for example, tuberculosis resulting in tuberculoma or bronchiectasis resulting in brain abscess, may have a similar significance.

Computerised tomographic (C.T.) scanning

Computerised tomography requires very expensive apparatus, but provides information of great value regarding the contents of the skull. The investigation is safe and painless. The ventricular system and cortical sulci are displayed. Areas of cortical atrophy may be seen (Fig. 26). Neoplasms are shown by virtue of their altered X-ray absorption relative to that of the surrounding normal brain (Fig. 27). Radiological contrast media may be injected intravenously and will leak into areas in

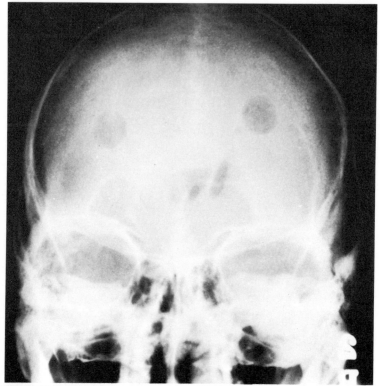

Fig. 29 Shift of ventricular system.

which the blood-brain barrier is defective (e.g. neoplasms, abscesses, areas of infarction). Such areas of increased uptake of contrast medium are readily detected by C.T. scanning.

Pneumoencephalography

Pneumoencephalography (air encephalography, A.E.G.) has passed into very limited use where C.T. scanning is available. Air encephalography provides much the same type of information as C.T. scanning in relation to the configuration of the ventricular system and the cortical surface (Fig. 28), and yields clearer pictures. It provides C.S.F. for examination, but it will not display the dimensions of lesions within the brain substance, as C.T. scanning does.

Ventriculography

Ventriculography, outlining as it does the ventricular system, supplies much the same information as air encephalography but it can be utilised in two additional situations.

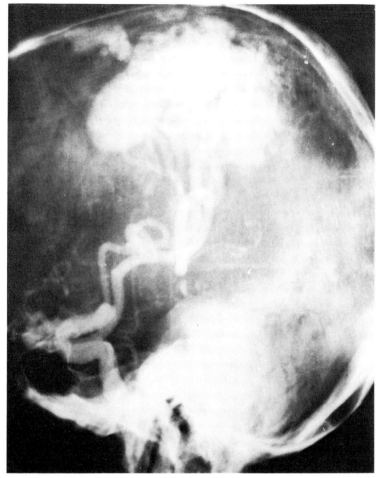

Fig. 30 Angiogram showing an arteriovenous malformation in the parietal lobe. In this arterial phase the abnormal vessels of the malformation are seen, including veins of very large diameter which fill unduly rapidly.

1. When intracranial pressure is obviously raised and air encephalography is therefore contraindicated.

2. When air introduced by the lumbar route fails to enter the ventricular system.

The procedure has the disadvantage that burr holes must be made in the skull and needles inserted through brain tissue. Fig. 29 illustrates shift of the ventricular system demonstrated by ventriculography.

Angiography
Angiography is of diagnostic value in three circumstances.

1. The investigation of intracranial space-occupying lesions (intra-

cerebral or extracerebral haematomata, abscesses, neoplasms) regardless of whether or not intracranial pressure is raised. Further, the vascular pattern of a neoplasm may provide some indication of its pathology.

2. The investigation of vascular abnormalities such as arteriovenous malformations and aneurysms (Fig. 30).

3. The investigation of cerebrovascular occlusive disease by demonstrating atherosclerotic changes, stenosis or occlusion of major vessels.

The investigation, however, is not without risk; for example, subintimal injection of contrast material may lead to occlusion of a major artery; embolism may result from injection of a blood clot or dislodgement of atheromatous material at the site of injection; arterial spasm may result from irritation produced by the contrast medium, or the patient may collapse due to hypersensitivity to the medium.

Radio-isotope (gamma) brain scanning

This investigation depends on the localised breakdowns of the blood-brain barrier which may occur in relation to a cerebral tumour and other local pathologies including cerebral abscess and vascular lesions. Following the administration of substances labelled with radio-isotopes (e.g. radio-isotope labelled human albumin), scanning of the brain may show an increased uptake of isotope in relation to the local pathology as compared with its surroundings.

Again this investigation is safe and painless and is widely used as a screening procedure in patients suspected of having a cerebral tumour. A negative scan does not necessarily exclude a supratentorial lesion and persisting focal E.E.G. abnormalities might with advantage be followed by serial scans at intervals until a tumour has been reasonably excluded. Radio-isotope scans are probably rather less useful than C.T. scans in investigating the cause of epilepsy. Both are likely to be successful in displaying tumours, but C.T. scanning can display atrophic lesions which may be the cause of epilepsy, while gamma scans cannot reveal such lesions.

ULTRASONIC ECHOENCEPHALOGRAPHY

This investigation, which is safe and painless, is used to detect lateral shift of midline structures. Although it lacks the diagnostic accuracy of air studies and angiography it has proved a useful screening measure for neoplasms of the cerebral hemispheres. Its use is diminishing with the wider availability of C.T. and radio-isotope brain scans.

LUMBAR PUNCTURE

On the whole, lumbar puncture and examination of the cerebrospinal fluid is of extremely limited value in the investigation of epilepsy and, although it has certain indications, it may also have definite dangers. Thus, although the risk of performing lumbar puncture in the presence of obviously raised intracranial pressure is well recognised, it is not unknown for lumbar puncture to be performed when a patient has had an epileptic seizure for the first time in adult life and when, therefore, an intracranial neoplasm enters into the differential diagnosis. In such instances the risk of uncal herniation and mid-brain compression as a result of withdrawal of cerebrospinal fluid, although significant, may not be adequately recognised, possibly because the effects of compression may not be apparent for several days and may then be attributed to the disease process rather than to this ancillary investigation.

Lumbar puncture should not be performed as a routine investigation of epilepsy but it may prove of value in the following circumstances:

1. Distinguishing between meningitis and subarachnoid haemorrhage.
2. Diagnosing the presence and type of meningitis.
3. Establishing the diagnosis of neurosyphilis.
4. Helping to establish the diagnosis of multiple sclerosis, subacute inclusion body encephalitis or 'infectious' polyneuritis.

BIOCHEMICAL INVESTIGATIONS

The relevant biochemical investigations are too numerous to mention in detail. They should be performed as indicated by the history and by the clinical picture and, in particular, serological tests for syphilis, prolonged fasting blood glucose estimations, tolbutamide tolerance tests or plasma insulin assays and estimations of serum calcium and blood urea may furnish information of great diagnostic value in the investigation of secondary epilepsy.

Clinical evaluation determines the pattern of subsequent ancillary investigations, but it must be emphasised that investigations such as C.T. scanning, angiography and air studies are not infallible. Particularly in early, slowly growing avascular tumours, which are too small to distort the ventricular system or displace blood vessels, these investigations may furnish negative or equivocal results. The fact that such investigations may have to be repeated later must be accepted.

INVESTIGATION IN PARTICULAR FORMS OF EPILEPSY

The decision as to how extensively to investigate the aetiology of epilepsy must be made in relation to the individual problem in every patient. However, some general guidelines can be suggested.

1. If the history suggests that the patient has a variety of *generalised epilepsy* and the family history is positive there may be no need to investigate past electroencephalography if this confirms the diagnosis. If the family history is negative, but the patient's seizure history and the E.E.G. are typical, there is probably also no need to investigate further, particularly if there is a story of birth difficulty or prematurity. In the small group of cases of generalised epilepsy who do not fit into the two categories discussed above it is usually best to adopt a wait and see policy once the E.E.G. is carried out. A few such cases may have a brain degeneration, but such conditions are generally untreatable and early diagnosis may offer no advantages.

2. If the story suggests the patient has *partial epilepsy*, investigation must be taken at least as far as an E.E.G. Unless there is a well defined and adequate cause of partial epilepsy apparent from the history, and unless the E.E.G. also shows only focal spike activity, investigation such as skull and chest X-ray and C.T. scanning need to be considered. Even if these investigations are negative, the patient should be kept under clinical and E.E.G. observation for several years. If the epilepsy proves difficult to control, or a focal abnormality in the E.E.G. worsens, C.T. scanning and other neuroradiological procedures may have to be repeated in case a hitherto occult tumour has become evident.

SUMMARY

1. Assessment of patient suspected of having epilepsy depends on the sequence:
history ⟶ clinical examination ⟶
differential diagnosis ⟶ ancillary investigations ⟶
precise diagnosis.

2. History ⟶
- Symptoms preceding seizure
- Precipitating factors
- Postictal phenomena
- Previous and family history
- Eye witness account of seizure

3. Clinical examination ⟶
- General appearance of patient
- General physical examination
- Full neurological examination

4. Ancillary investigations:

   a. Electroencephalography
   b. X-rays of skull and chest
   c. Echoencephalography
   d. C.T. scanning
   e. Radioisotope scanning
   f. Lumbar puncture and examination of C.S.F.

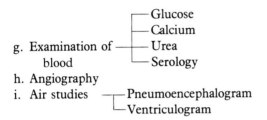

   g. Examination of ──┬── Glucose / Calcium / Urea / Serology
       blood
   h. Angiography
   i. Air studies ──┬── Pneumoencephalogram
                 └── Ventriculogram

FURTHER READING

Cala L A, Mastaglia F L, Woodings T L 1977 Computerised tomography of the cranium in patients with epilepsy: a preliminary report. Clin Exptl Neurol 14: 237

Du Boulay G H 1965 Principles of X-ray diagnosis of the skull. Butterworths, London

Eadie M J, Tyrer J H, Tod P A, Sutherland J M 1962 The diagnosis of tuberose sclerosis. Med J Aust 1: 547

Eadie M J, Sutherland J M, Tyrer J H 1963 The clinical features of hemifacial atrophy. Med J Aust 2: 177

Hill D 1963 Epilepsy: clinical aspects. In: Hill D, Parr G (ed) Electroencephalography, 2nd edn. Macdonald and Gee, London

Morley J B, Sephton R G 1969 The additional role of the scan in the diagnosis of cerebral tumours. Proc Australian Ass Neurol 6: 145

Plantiol T 1966 Some aspects of brain investigation by means of radio isotopes. J Neurol Sci 3: 539

Robertson E G 1967 Pneumoencephalography, 2nd edn. Charles C Thomas, Springfield

Sutherland J M, Eadie M J, Mann P R, Tyrer J H 1966 Ancillary investigations in neurological diagnosis. Med J Aust 2: 542

Taveras J M, Wood E H 1964 Diagnostic Neuroradiology. Williams & Wilkins Co, Baltimore

6

The treatment of epilepsy

The treatment of patients with epilepsy is not only a matter of drug therapy. Effective management depends initially on an accurate and comprehensive diagnosis of the type of epilepsy and of its cause. It is not sufficient to diagnose 'epilepsy' and prescribe an anticonvulsant drug. If the correct diagnosis is 'generalised epilepsy', it should be determined whether this is hereditary ('primary') or due to structural or chemical pathology. Further, the type of generalised epilepsy should be determined (tonic-clonic seizures, myoclonic attacks, petit mal absences, or a combination of these) since this qualification has a therapeutic and prognostic significance. If, on the other hand, the diagnosis is 'partial (symptomatic) epilepsy', the underlying pathology should be assessed and, if possible, treated while controlling the seizures with appropriate anticonvulsant therapy.

Adequate treatment of the patient with epilepsy must comprise his total care and not merely the treatment of his seizures. Patients and relatives should be informed as to how they may best deal with individual seizures, and the doctor should be prepared to advise on various difficulties which may arise in the course of an 'epileptic's' life. To do this adequately the doctor should be aware of the patient's and his family's attitude to the diagnosis of epilepsy, of how the local community is likely to regard the disorder and of what opportunities there are locally for education and employment. Every doctor undertaking the management of patients suffering from epilepsy should have a knowledge of the indications and limitations of available anticonvulsant drugs as well as their possible side effects, and the complications of epilepsy itself. Finally, the physician should be aware of the possibility of neurosurgical treatment in selected cases of epilepsy.

THE MANAGEMENT OF A PATIENT WITH EPILEPSY

This comprises the following six aspects:

1. Adequate assessment and diagnosis.

2. The treatment of individual seizures when necessary (see below).
3. An appreciation of, and advice on various general and social implications (see below).
4. Anticonvulsant therapy (Ch. 7).
5. The treatment of complications, including status epilepticus (Ch. 8).
6. Consideration of the role of neurosurgery in epilepsy (Ch. 9).

THE TREATMENT OF AN EPILEPTIC SEIZURE

To the layman, a major epileptic seizure is frightening to witness but only rarely does the patient come to harm. It is important to emphasise this to parents or relatives who may be called on to deal with a seizure, and to advise them what to do in such an event.

1. The patient should be gently restrained to avoid injuring himself by striking hard objects or burning or drowning himself.

2. If the patient is unconscious a clear airway should be maintained by turning him onto his side, and by holding his lower jaw forwards. This can be accomplished only when the patient has reached the flaccid stage of the seizure. Unprotected fingers should not be inserted into the patient's mouth. Usually the clonic stage has been reached before any action to prevent tongue biting can be taken though sometimes in the tonic phase a rolled up portion of towel or a handkerchief can be inserted into the angle of the mouth to act as a gag. Teeth have been broken by overenthusiastic attempts to introduce pegs or handles of spoons as gags. (Parents and relatives of patients with epilepsy should be advised that broken teeth are a greater problem than a bitten tongue and that almost always there is no need to do anything at all about maintaining a clear airway as the patient recovers from the seizure without any treatment.)

3. If a second seizure follows without consciousness being regained, it is generally advisable to summon medical advice because of the risk of status epilepticus developing. Otherwise there is no need for urgent medical attention unless the patient remains unconscious for more than a few minutes after the seizure has ended.

4. In seizures characterised by disturbed behaviour without convulsions the patient should be handled with persuasion and gentle restraint. Such patients may react violently to other than gentle physical restriction.

5. In simple absences and other minor seizures there is generally no need to take any action at all other than to maintain a watch on the patient until he appears normal again.

GENERAL AND SOCIAL IMPLICATIONS

In epilepsy, as in most other conditions, total patient care is essential. The proper care of a patient with epilepsy is comprehensive and in addition to adequate drug therapy, the patient's psychological difficulties must be appreciated and his fears overcome by discussion and counselling; his economic and occupational status may require evaluation; special circumstances, such as marriage or pregnancy, require individual consideration.

Unfortunately there is still a considerable amount of lay ignorance tinged with superstitious beliefs regarding epilepsy. Whereas many other conditions excite sympathy, epilepsy is still not quite socially acceptable, and may even produce rejection and revulsion. In a series of 160 consecutive epileptic outpatients attending Royal Brisbane Hospital, Edwards (1974) found that 58 per cent considered that their social life had been impaired by having epilepsy. A diagnosis of epilepsy tends to be equated with mental disorder and employers tend to categorise patients with epilepsy as being substandard employees. Certainly, as in any other disorder, co-existent impairment of intellect or personality disorder may be present in persons with epilepsy, and in a minority of patients deterioration of personality (possibly related to organic neuronal damage produce by seizures or drug overdosage) may develop. Further, some children with petit mal absences may display neurotic tendencies, and temporal lobe epilepsy may correlate with aggressive or otherwise disturbed behaviour. In general, however, it should be emphasised that there is no consistent relationship between epilepsy and intelligence or behaviour.

Epilepsy may lead to the patient's feeling 'different' or 'set apart' from his fellows. There is a wish to forget that he is 'an epileptic' and this in turn may lead to rejection or omission of drug therapy. Of the 160 patients referred to above, 18 per cent were resentful at having epilepsy but proved cooperative while a further 6 per cent tended to reject the diagnosis and would not adhere to regular drug therapy. Further seizures may lead to loss of employment, difficulty in obtaining employment, or change to a lower level of employment. In other patients anxiety regarding marriage, pregnancy and the development of epilepsy in their children may be present. Such factors tend to engender feelings of inferiority and sometimes lead to paranoid thought patterns in the patient with epilepsy.

Children with epilepsy may be psychologically rejected by their parents who, however, compensate for this by a display of overprotection. The neurotic traits of personality disorders which may be associated with epilepsy can produce tension in the home or school environment and lead to deterioration in parent–child or teacher–child relationships, a deterioration which becomes more intense if the child belongs to an unstable family unit.

In our view, it is generally wise to have a frank discussion with the patient or, if a child, with the parents regarding the nature of epilepsy. It can be emphasised that epilepsy is not a disease but rather a symptom of disturbed electrical activity in the brain. In 'generalised, (primary) epilepsy', the concept of a seizure threshold may help the patient, or parent, to appreciate that every brain is potentially epileptic though in some people this tendency is greater than in others. Drug treatment is designed to normalise the threshold for seizures and, thus, to protect the patient until, perhaps, a normal seizure threshold is achieved by the processes of nature and suppression of abnormal (seizure) activity.

In partial (symptomatic) epilepsy the lay person may readily understand how a local 'short circuit' may result in a focal seizure and will gain reassurance from the analogy that, if there has also been a major seizure, this is simply due to the short circuit 'overloading' the brain stem 'fuse box'.

Reassurance should also be given that epilepsy when controlled does not lead to any mental disorder or intellectual deterioration. Advice can be given that patients with epilepsy should lead a normal well balanced life with only certain commonsense restrictions. Thus, there is no dietary restriction; if desired, patients can drink alcohol in moderation unless their seizures are known to follow alcohol intake. Some 16 per cent Edwards' (1974) series considered alcohol a precipitating factor. Patients may also take part in the majority of sports and recreational activities.

Certain age groups may require specific counselling.

SPECIFIC COUNSELLING

Schooling
Some 80 per cent of children who develop seizures after infancy are intellectually normal. These children should attend a normal school and be educated to the limit of their potential in the usual way. Over-excitement and over-fatigue may be best avoided for some but the child should play games and take part in all the usual school activities. Certain activities such as swimming must be carefully supervised. It is wise for the parents to inform the school authorities and the school medical officer of the child's condition and to enlist the school teacher's cooperation and interest, particularly if there is any tendency to behavioural or other psychological difficulties. In our opinion, from

a scholastic point of view, many children with appropriate types of epilepsy are better when treated with phenytoin (Dilantin) than with phenobarbitone, which because of its general sedative effects on brain function may lower effective intelligence. Additionally pheno-barbitone not infrequently, paradoxically, increases tendencies to emotional instability and aggressiveness.

Career planning

Apart from instances of typical benign febrile convulsions in infancy, children or adolescents with a past history of any form of epilepsy should be advised that they will not be able to obtain a licence to pilot an aeroplane, and that they should avoid occupations involving the driving of public transport. When an adolescent with incompletely controlled epilepsy is likely to enter the workforce in the next two or three years, he should be counselled against seeking employment in which he may have to work on heights or near open machinery or fire or in which his future prospects will depend on his being able to drive a car. At times such advice may prove unnecessarily cautious, but it is better not to let the subject proceed too far along a career which becomes closed once epilepsy has occurred again.

Occupation

If the epileptic state is fully controlled by anticonvulsant therapy over a period of two or three years, the patient can undertake almost any type of employment he or she is otherwise capable of, apart from driving public transport (passenger vehicles, locomotives or aircraft). If, however, occasional attacks occur, advice regarding occupation has to be individualised with particular reference to working at heights, with electricity or machinery, or where there is potential danger to the patient or others should he develop a seizure. In some instances rehabilitation may be necessary to fit the individual for some alternative type of employment.

Regrettably, because of the uninformed attitude of many employers to epilepsy, it is our custom at times to advise some patients not to divulge the fact that they suffer from epilepsy unless specifically questioned. The importance of assisting the patient with regard to occupation is emphasised by Edwards' (1974) findings. In his series of 160 patients, approximately 20 per cent were classed as invalid pensioners. Of 76 employable individuals 38 per cent gave a history of having been refused employment when the history of epilepsy was disclosed, while 59 per cent had elected to conceal this history from their employers. Thirty-two per cent of the patients who had disclosed the diagnosis considered that they had been well treated by their employers, while 44 per cent believed that their careers had been compromised in significant degree.

Car driving

This is largely a matter of social conscience. In Edwards' series, 118 patients were of an age to hold a driving licence. Twenty-six patients, indeed, held a licence and of those 21 were not regarded as being adequately controlled, having had a seizure within the previous two years. The ability to drive a motor vehicle is an important skill in our civilisation and the loss of a licence to drive may lead to loss of earnings, unemployment and hardship with consequent increase in feelings of being discriminated against. On the other hand, patients with poorly controlled epileptic seizures, when driving a car, constitute a hazard to themselves and others. In some countries including Australia, it is not the doctor's duty to inform the appropriate authorities that a patient has epilepsy or should not be allowed to drive, but in such instances the doctor should do all in his power to persuade the patient (or the patient's family) that, at the present time, the patient should not drive a motor vehicle. It is obvious that, although logical and correct, such advice may lead to feelings of discrimination and be regarded by the patient as a punitive measure. To mitigate these reactions, it should be indicated that the advice to discontinue driving is subject to review provided that the patient cooperates by taking anticonvulsant medicines and remains seizure free over a period of some years.

The legal position. This appears to vary from country to country. In some, a patient with epilepsy can obtain a licence to drive if he has been free of seizures for two to three years even if he is still taking anticonvulsant drugs. In at least one other, it was held that if the patient is taking anticonvulsant drugs to control seizures he must still, in law, be suffering from epilepsy and cannot therefore hold a driving licence.

Medical advice. Bearing in mind the foregoing, from a medical point of view each patient must be given individual consideration. Medical opinion on this question varies from country to country and within countries from doctor to doctor; but in our opinion, provided the patient has had no epileptic seizures over a period of at least three years, it would seem, in general, reasonable to permit him to hold a driving licence, particularly if the electroencephalogram has reverted to normal and provided he abstains from alcohol before driving. In these patients, there is a reasonable basis for concluding that the individual is no longer suffering from epilepsy. It will be apparent that patients who have only had nocturnal epileptic seizures merit special consideration. Since anticonvulsant therapy helps to keep patients seizure-free, and since phenytoin in average dosage does not affect driving skill, there is something to be said for continuing pheyntoin therapy over an indefinite period of years.

If it is decided, however, to discontinue anticonvulsant therapy, the patient should be discouraged from driving during the period of drug reduction and for 12 months after the drug is ceased, because of the enhanced risk of seizures during this time.

The armed services
Despite the well attested historical fact that Julius Caesar suffered from epilepsy, a history of epilepsy generally debars the individual from service with the Armed Forces.

Insurance
Most insurance companies are willing to consider each case on its merits. Generally, the applicant should be free of seizures for at least two years but with the exception of epilepsy occurring secondary to a progressive pathology, a policy may be offered though often subject to 'loading' which will vary in accordance with the medical evidence of the risks.

Marriage and genetic problems
Advice as to whether a patient suffering from epilepsy should marry must depend on the individual patient. In both primary and secondary epilepsy, the prospective marriage partner should be informed by the patient of the position and it is often helpful for the doctor to see both the patient and the prospective partner together so that the position can be fully explained and any questions answered.

In *generalised epilepsy*, two factors merit consideration:

1. the severity of the epilepsy and
2. genetic factors.

If, for example, the epileptic state is a severe one in that control has proved impossible to achieve or if there is evidence of intellectual or personality deterioration, marriage may be contraindicated as in any other serious condition. In lesser degrees of epilepsy, there is no reason to advise against marriage; it can be stated that the epilepsy will be made neither worse nor better by the married state.

With regard to genetic factors, the trait appears to be transmitted as an autosomal dominant with a variable degree of penetrance. There is, therefore, a 50 per cent risk that the offspring of a parent with this type of epilepsy will have a tendency to generalised epilepsy although this may not result in clinical epilepsy in their lifetimes. If both parents have hereditary generalised epilepsy, the risk of transmitting the disorder and of clinical epilepsy occurring in the progeny is naturally much higher.

In *generalised epilepsy due to structural or chemical pathology* and in *partial epilepsy (i.e. symptomatic epilepsies)*, advice given will depend largely on the underlying pathology. If it is due to one of the heredofamilial disorders the risk of the epilepsy being transmitted is that of the primary disease. If, however, the pathological condition has been acquired (e.g. trauma or encephalitis), genetic factors are of little or no significance. The risk of epilepsy in the offspring is as for any other member of the general population.

Advice may be sought by parents who have one child with epilepsy and who fear that other children they may have will be similarly affected. The answer to such a query will depend on the type of epilepsy the affected child suffers from and, if a family history exists, on the nature of the epilepsy in either or both parents. If the child has symptomatic epilepsy due, for example, to birth trauma, and if there is no family history of epilepsy, the risk of subsequent children having epilepsy is that of the incidence of the condition in the general population (so long as the mother does not have some obstetric abnormality which predisposes her children to brain damage at birth). If, on the other hand, the child's epileptic state is primary (hereditary) in type, advice given will depend on a consideration of the genetic factors already discussed.

Pregnancy
Epilepsy may occur in relation to pregnancy in the following ways:

1. Generalised or partial epilepsy may occur for the first time during pregnancy.
2. Pregnancy may activate epilepsy (generalised or partial) which has been latent for many years.
3. Pregnancy may lead to increase of vascularity or even to change in the cytology of a meningioma and thus lead to the appearance of focal cerebral signs, including epilepsy.
4. Eclampsia may occasion a metabolic disturbance associated with cerebral vasoconstriction. Under these circumstances epileptic seizures may occur—an extracranial secondary type of epilepsy, generalised or partial.
5. In the puerperium, epileptic seizures may develop and have been ascribed to vascular lesions, particularly in a temporal lobe.

In an individual patient who has previously suffered from epilepsy, it is not possible to predict the effect of pregnancy on the epilepsy. The metabolic changes associated with pregnancy (particularly excess weight gain due to overhydration and sodium retention) would favour an increased tendency to seizures, and it has been estimated that an increased number of attacks will occur in about one third to one half of patients with epilepsy during their pregnancy. However recent work has shown that there is an increased requirement for anticonvulsant drugs during pregnancy. Unless drug doses are increased during pregnancy plasma and brain levels of the drugs fall, and anti-epileptic effect diminishes. Since this phenomenon has been recognised and anticonvulsant doses have been adjusted during pregnancy to maintain plasma anticonvulsant levels at pre-pregnancy values, the writers have the impression that there has been very little tendency for epilepsy to worsen during pregnancy in their patients.

Maternal intake of phenytoin, phenobarbitone and probably other anticonvulsants appears to be associated with a small risk of teratogenic effects. However, it is not completely established that it is taking the drugs, rather than having epilepsy, which is responsible for the occurrence of the malformations. There has been a report of macrocytic anaemia and thrombocytopaenia occurring in a baby whose mother had been taking these drugs but this occurrence must be very rare. A bleeding tendency has occurred in neonates born to mothers who took anticonvulsants during pregnancy. This tendency can be prevented by injecting the mother with vitamin K during labour.

The law on termination of pregnancy. This varies substantialy from place to place. In some countries this procedure may be carried out only to preserve the life of the mother. Its justifiable use will then be uncommon, as in those patients who are likely to have a severe status epilepticus precipitated by the pregnancy and who have a past history indicating that such a status would quite possibly be uncontrollable.

In Britain, the Abortions Act increased substantially the legal indications for termination of pregnancy and probably applies where there is a substantial risk of the child inheriting, for example, a neuro-lipoidosis.

Travel

In assessing medical fitness of the patient with epilepsy for international travel, consideration must be given to the effects of disturbed sleep, exhaustion, climatic changes, effects of intercurrent illnesses which may be contracted and the degree of control of the seizures. Little exception could be taken to a patient with well controlled epilepsy undertaking a short flight or a leisurely sea voyage on a ship carrying a ship's surgeon, whereas at the other end of the scale, one would advise against a patient with poorly controlled epilepsy travelling a long distance by air. Between these extremes, other patients must be assessed according to all the circumstances.

SUMMARY

1. The management of an epileptic patient

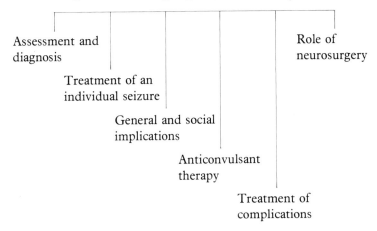

Assessment and diagnosis

Treatment of an individual seizure

General and social implications

Anticonvulsant therapy

Treatment of complications

Role of neurosurgery

2. General social implications

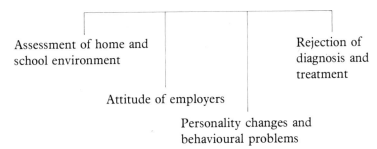

Assessment of home and school environment

Attitude of employers

Personality changes and behavioural problems

Rejection of diagnosis and treatment

3. Specific counselling

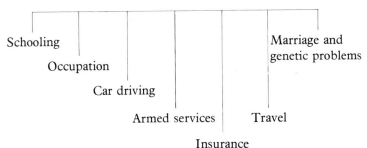

Schooling

Occupation

Car driving

Armed services

Insurance

Travel

Marriage and genetic problems

4. Pregnancy and epilepsy

a. Generalised or partial epilepsy may occur for first time during pregnancy.

b. Pregnancy may activate latent epilepsy.

c. Pregnancy may increase vascularity in a meningioma ⟶ focal signs ± epilepsy.

d. Pregnancy may cause eclampsia ⟶ cerebral oedema and cerebral vasoconstriction ⟶ secondary (intracranial) epilepsy.

e. In puerperium, an intracranial vascular lesion may lead to epilepsy.

f. Epilepsy may rarely be an indication for termination of pregnancy.

g. Epilepsy may not worsen during pregnancy if anticonvulsant drug doses are adjusted to meet the increased dosage requirement of pregnancy.

FURTHER READING

Edwards V E 1974 Social problems confronting a person with epilepsy in modern society. Proc Aust Assoc Neurol 11: 239
Espir M L E 1967 Epilepsy and driving. Lancet 1: 375
Janz D 1975 The teratogenic risk of antiepileptic drugs. Epilepsia 16: 159–169
Knight A H, Rhind E G 1975 Epilepsy and pregnancy: a study of 153 pregnancies in 59 patients. Epilepsia 16: 99
Lander C M, Edwards V E, Eadie M J, Tyrer J H 1977 Plasma anticonvulsant concentrations during pregnancy. Neurology (Minneap) 27: 128
Livingstone S 1972 Comprehensive management of epilepsy in infancy, childhood and adolescence. Charles C Thomas, Springfield
Taylor D C 1971 Prevention in epileptic disorders. Lancet 2: 1136

7

Anticonvulsant drug therapy

Although the use of bromide has now been abandoned, effective medical treatment for epileptic seizures dates from the introduction of this drug in 1857. Since this time, a large number of anticonvulsant drugs has become available yet medical treatment of epilepsy still falls short of the ideal. With efficient therapy adequate seizure control can be achieved in some 70 to 80 per cent of patients. Unwanted effects of drug therapy, however, are not uncommon and a number of patients' epilepsies remain resistant to any drug, or drug combination, available at the present time.

ANTICONVULSANT DISPOSITION

With the exception of sodium valproate (a branched chain fatty acid) the currently available anticonvulsant drugs are heterocyclic compounds, several of which contain fairly similar five or six membered ring structures with a variety of substituent groups. In most patients the anticonvulsants appear to be virtually fully absorbed from the alimentary tract though there is suspicion that carbamazepine may sometimes absorb incompletely. After absorption they are distributed through the various tissues and body fluids (Fig. 31) but there appears to be relatively little, if any, selective regional concentration of the drugs in the brain. Many of the anticonvulsants are present in plasma, in part bound to plasma protein, and in part free in plasma water. However primidone and ethosuximide appear not to bind to plasma proteins. The anticonvulsant drug in plasma water is in equilibrium with the drug in the brain, and is also in equilibrium with any of the drug that is bound to plasma protein. The biological effects of an anticonvulsant are related to its concentration at its sites of action in the brain. The concentration of the drug in plasma water or, less directly but more conveniently, in whole plasma, is therefore a measure of its brain concentration and its biological activity.

Anticonvulsant drugs are metabolised in the liver. Some e.g., methylphenobarbitone, primidone, trimethadione, form initial meta-

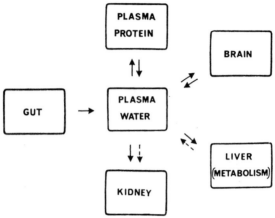

Fig. 31 Pattern of drug distribution.

bolites with anticonvulsant activities approximately equal to those of the parent drugs, but further metabolism occurs so that the anticonvulsants are finally converted to compounds which have very little or no biological activity. These are excreted in the urine as such, or conjugated with glucuronic or sulphuric acids. Some unmetabolised anticonvulsant also may appear in the urine.

The liver's rate of metabolising anticonvulsants varies considerably from person to person, but usually is slow enough for plasma and brain concentrations of the drug to remain relatively constant over the dosage interval if the drug is taken once or twice daily. When anticonvulsant treatment is begun, or anticonvulsant doses are changed, it usually requires several days for plasma and brain levels of the drug to reach a steady state. In the steady state mean plasma levels of a drug remains constant from one dosage interval to the next. The main factors governing tissue levels of an anticonvulsant are the dosage in which the drug is given, and the liver's rate of metabolising the drug. The latter can be altered in liver disease, and a congenital deficiency in the liver's metabolising enzyme system has been described at least in relation to phenytoin. Anticonvulsant metabolism may be altered by the intake of other drugs. Many such interactions have been reported. Some of the more important ones are set out in Table 7 but the list is not exhaustive. It seems likely that further such interactions will be found as time passes. The various circumstances which can alter anticonvulsant metabolism point to the necessity for reviewing anticonvulsant dosage in the presence of liver disease, or if other drugs are given simultaneously. There is also evidence that, in uraemia, the plasma protein bindings of phenytoin and other drugs are altered. Less drug is bound to plasma protein than in the normal man, so that

Table 7   The more important pharmacokinetic interactions affecting the major anticonvulsants

Anticonvulsant	Drugs raising plasma levels of the Anticonvulsant	Drugs lowering plasma levels of the Anticonvulsant
Phenytoin	Sulthiame; ethosuximide; valproate[a]; dicumarol; sulphonamides; isoniazid[a]; prochlorperazine	carbamazepine[a]: clonazepam[a]; folic acid;
Carbamazepine	propoxyphene;	phenytoin; phenobarbitone;
Phenobarbitone	phenytoin; valproate;	—
Ethosuximide	—	
Clonazepam	—	phenytoin; phenobarbitone
Valproate	—	?phenytoin; phenobarbitone

[a]These interactions are known to be inconstant. Some of the other interactions have not been studied in enough subjects to be sure that they are consistently present.

biological effects (which are related to the concentration of the drug in plasma water) occur at lower total plasma drug levels than would be expected.

MECHANISM OF ANTICONVULSANT ACTION

At the present time the mechanism of action of the anticonvulsant drugs is incompletely understood and no general theory of anticonvulsant action is possible. As will be explained shortly, different chemical families of anticonvulsants have relatively specific actions against different types of epilepsy in man, and also against different types of experimental epilepsy. Of the two classical tests for the anticonvulsant activity of a drug in the experimental animal (electroshock induced seizures and pentylenetetrazole induced seizures), drugs of value in major epilepsy e.g. phenytoin, tend to protect against the former, whereas drugs useful in petit mal absences e.g., troxidone, tend to protect against the latter. Some drugs e.g., methsuximide (Celontin) may have activity against both types of seizure.

A number of biochemical effects of the anticonvulsants which could help protect against epilepsy are known. For example phenytoin decreases intraneuronal Na^+ concentrations, though the way in which this effect is produced is uncertain. The consequent increased Na^+ gradient across the neuronal cell membrane should tend to make the neurone less excitable and diminishes the likelihood of post-tetanic hyperpolarisation of the nerve terminal and post-tetanic potentiation. Troxidone is metabolised in the liver to an acid substance (dimethadione). If this produces an intraneuronal acidosis the increased hydrogen ion concentration within the neurone may lead to an increased potential difference across the neuronal cell membrane, and to lessened excitability of the neurone. Several anticonvulsants e.g. the barbiturates, can inhibit the terminal stages of mitochondrial oxidation processes, so that the neurone may not have sufficient energy available to form synaptic transmitter substances in adequate quantities. However, this effect tends to occur at higher drug concentrations than those likely to be produced during anticonvulsant therapy in man. Therapy with several anticonvulsants may lead to a state of folate deficiency, but there is no proof that anticonvulsant effect is due to lack of folate in the neurone. Several anticonvulsants alter brain concentrations of the synaptic transmitters noradrenaline and serotonin, while valproate increases brain levels of the inhibitory neurotransmitter gamma aminobutyric acid (GABA).

ANTICONVULSANT SIDE EFFECTS

Apart from *local irritative effects* at their site of administration e.g. nausea, anticonvulsant side effects tend to fall into three categories:
  1. *Idiosyncrasy or hypersensitivity effects,* most commonly involving the skin but sometimes involving the blood forming organs and other tissues e.g., the kidney.
  2. *Dosage related effects.* These vary from drug to drug and may involve various organs, but in excessive dosage all the anticonvulsants tend to produce drowsiness and unsteadiness.
  3. *Effects on the foetus and neonate.* Recently it has been shown that the risk of congenital malformation in the children of epileptic mothers treated with phenytoin or phenobarbitone is about double that of children of non-epileptic mothers. However, it has not been shown conclusively whether this is due to the treatment, or to the epilepsy itself. The use of anticonvulsants in pregnancy may accelerate the metabolism of vitamin K, causing a bleeding tendency in the new born.

ADJUSTMENT OF ANTICONVULSANT DOSAGE

Anticonvulsant metabolism varies so much from person to person that only general guidelines to drug dosage can be given. There is a natural tendency to recommend doses on the low side of the average effective dose. It is essential to realise that effective doses, and toxic doses of the same drug, vary greatly from patient to patient. If an anticonvulsant dose does not control epilepsy in a patient the dose should be increased until the epilepsy is stopped, or until side effects prevent further dosage increases. In general there should be no predetermined upper or lower limit of dose. If facilities exist, plasma anticonvulsant levels can be measured and the results used as a guide to dosage changes.

Such measurements permit dose-related adverse effects to be detected at an early stage, and also may reveal failures of compliance with the prescribed anticonvulsant regime.

As mentioned earlier, the effects of anticonvulsants are related to drug concentrations in brain, and this is in turn related to drug concentrations in plasma. For several anticonvulsants ranges of plasma drug levels have been found which offer the best chance of controlling epilepsy, with a minimal risk of overdosage effects. These ranges are referred to as the 'therapeutic ranges' but it should be understood that, in the individual, epilepsy may be controlled with plasma anticonvulsant levels above or below the 'therapeutic' range. Therapeutic ranges of the anticonvulsants, and average dose to produce plasma drug levels in the therapeutic range for each drug, are shown in Table 8. In adjusting phenytoin doses to attain concentrations in the therapeutic range it should be realised that equal dosage increments produce increasingly rapid rates of rise in plasma phenytoin level, as the level itself increases (Fig. 32). If this is not appreciated unexpected overdosage may occur. This effect is not so noticeable with phenobarbitone and ethosuximide, but does occur.

The ability to measure plasma anticonvulsant levels, and to adjust doses in terms of these levels, is particularly important in types of epilepsy in which seizures recur only at long intervals. When seizures occur frequently, as in petit mal absences, it is easier to adjust drug doses on the basis of clinical response only.

THE CHOICE OF AN ANTICONVULSANT DRUG

Experience has shown that particular anticonvulsant drugs are most

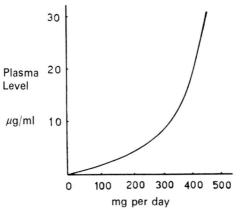

Fig. 32 The disproportionate increase in steady-state plasma phenytoin level which occurs when phenytoin dose is increased in the individual patient.

likely to be useful in particular types of epilepsy. Thus correct identification of type of epilepsy is a prerequisite for successful anticonvulsant drug therapy. The correlation between type of epilepsy and potentially suitable drugs is as shown in Table 9.

Table 8 Therapeutic ranges of anticonvulsants, and typical dosages to achieve plasma levels in the therapeutic range

Drug	Plasma therapeutic range		Usual dose[a] (mg/kg/day)
	μG/ml	μM/litre	
Phenytoin (Dilantin: Epanutin)	10–20	40–80	{ 5 (adults); 8 (children)
Carbamazepine (Tegretol)	6–12	25–50	10–20
Phenobarbitone	10–30	45–130	{ 2 (adults); 4 (children)
Methylphenobarbitone (Prominal)	10–30 } as pheno- 10–30 } barbitone	45–130 } as pheno- barbitone	{ 5 (adults); 7 (children)
Primidone (Mysoline)		45–130	10
Ethosuximide (Zarontin)	40–120	300–900	30
Clonazepam (Rivotril)	0.025–0.075	0.075–0.200	0.1–0.2
Sodium valproate (Epilim)	50–100	300–600	20

[a]The relation between plasma drug level and dose varies considerably from patient to patient. Therefore, these figures can serve only as a rough guide to appropriate dosage.

Table 9

Type of epilepsy	First choice drugs	Second choice drugs
Generalised epilepsy		
1. *Absences*	ethosuximide; clonazepam; valproate	troxidone; phensuximide; methsuximide
2. *Myoclonic absences*		
(i) infantile spasms	corticotrophin; tetracosactrin; corticosteroids	valproate
(ii) Lennox-Gastaut syndrome	valproate; clonazepam	nitrazepam; ethosuximide; barbiturates
(iii) in adolescence	valproate; clonazepam; barbiturates	carbamazepine
3. *Tonic-clonic seizures*	barbiturates; valproate	carbamazepine, phenytoin; clonazepam
Partial epilepsy (without or with secondary tonic-clonic seizures)	phenytoin; carbamazepine; barbiturates	clonazepam; sulthiame; valproate; methoin

ANTICONVULSANT COMBINATIONS

Should an appropriate anticonvulsant drug be prescribed for a patient's epilepsy, and the dose be increased to the patients' limit of tolerance without fully controlling the seizures, it may be necessary to select a second appropriate anticonvulsant and give it in combination with the first drug. Once anticonvulsants are combined, interactions between the two drugs may occur. These can be detected by plasma drug level monitoring, and appropriate dosage adjustments can be made. Sometimes two drugs, each given in maximally tolerated doses, may fail to control epilepsy, and a third appropriate drug may have to be added. However, it should be pointed out that, if a patients' epilepsy has not been too long established before therapy is begun, in the majority of instances a single appropriate anticonvulsant will control all seizures, particularly when plasma drug level monitoring is used as a guide to optimal dosage from the outset of therapy.

DURATION OF ANTICONVULSANT THERAPY

In most forms of epilepsy it appears that if the patient can be kept completely free of seizures for three to five years, and if paroxysmal activity disappears from the E.E.G., there is a reasonable prospect that therapy can be withdrawn without the epilepsy recurring. If epilepsy cannot be fully controlled it is nearly always necessary to continue optimal anticonvulsant therapy indefinitely.

CLINICAL PHARMACOLOGY OF THE ANTICONVULSANT DRUGS

The pharmacology of the more important currently available anticonvulsants is dealt with below. The more frequently used groups of drugs are dealt with first, and at greater length.

HYDANTOIN ANTICONVULSANTS

Phenytoin or diphenylhydantoin (Dilantin: Epanutin) was first introduced in 1938. Experience which has accumulated since that time has confirmed the drug as being the most useful single anticonvulsant at present available for the treatment of partial epilepsy of all types. It is also useful in generalised epilepsy, apart from myoclonic seizures and petit mal absences.

The hydantoin most widely used, and probably the anticonvulsant most widely used, at the present time, is phenytoin. This drug will, therefore, be discussed at some length.

Phenytoin—diphenylhydantoin (Dilantin: Epanutin)

Phenytoin is often regarded as the drug of first choice in the control of tonic-clonic (major) epilepsy whether of primary generalised type or occurring due to secondary generalisation of partial seizures. Many would consider it the drug of first choice in all forms of epilepsy except petit mal or myoclonic attacks. However, the impression is growing that it may not be as effective as phenobarbitone in controlling tonic-clonic seizures of *primary* generalised epilepsy (including febrile convulsions). Although in partial epilepsy symptoms of the focal cortical discharge may sometimes be controlled, in other instances, even though major seizures due to a *secondary* generalisation of the partial discharge are prevented by phenytoin, the manifestations of the focal cortical discharge may continue. In such patients a combination of phenytoin and sulthiame (Ospolot) or carbamazepine (Tegretol), or phenobarbitone may prove effective.

The mode of action of phenytoin is not fully understood. The drug appears to inhibit the spread of seizure discharges rather than prevent their initiation. Whether it reduces neuronal excitability by decreasing intracellular sodium concentration is argued at present. Its effects occur particularly on synaptic transmission between neurones which discharge repetitively.

Side effects

Although a considerable number of side effects of phenytoin therapy have been reported, this is more a reflection on the widespread use of drug rather than on its high toxicity since it is, on the whole, a very safe drug.

The following side effects may occur:

Local effects. 1. Gastric upset is occasionally caused by the alkalinity of the sodium salt and may be encountered in the early days of treatment. It can be prevented by taking the drug with meals or with milk.

Idiosyncratic effects. 1. Dermatitis, a hypersensitivity reaction, occasionally occurs and may be accompanied by fever, eosinophilia, lymphadenopathy and, rarely, hepatitis.

2. Systemic lupus erythematosus has occurred rarely.

3. Gum hypertrophy results from the excessive deposition of

collagen. This occurs particularly in children and can be minimised by scrupulous dental hygiene. There is now some evidence that this symptom may be dose-related.

4. Hirsutism may develop, particularly on the limbs, and may prove a social embarrassment to female patients.

5. Occasional blood disturbances which have been reported include leucopenia, agranulocytosis, thrombocytopenia and aplastic anaemia.

6. Lymphadenopathy. This is a rare complication of phenytoin therapy. It may follow hypersensitivity dermatitis. The cervical nodes are usually most obviously affected but generalised lymphadenopathy associated with enlargement of liver and spleen may occur. More rarely, lymphadenopathy may be associated with pyrexia and atypical lymphocytes in the peripheral blood. A diagnosis of Hodgkin's disease or infectious mononucleosis may be suggested by the clinical picture and even a lymph node biopsy may be misleading. However, discontinuance of phenytoin therapy is useful both diagnostically and therapeutically since regression of the lymphadenopathy ensues within a week or two of withdrawing the drug. A malignant lymphadenopathy has occasionally been associated with phenytoin therapy.

Dose related side effects. 1. Cerebellar disturbance. A syndrome of cerebellar dysfunction appears to be related to the plasma concentration of phenytoin. Nystagmus develops at concentrations of about 20 μG/ml and ataxia of gait at concentrations of between 30 and 40 μG/ml. At higher plasma phenytoin levels drowsiness occurs. A slight degree of nystagmus and ataxia is, therefore, not infrequently produced as therapeutic levels of phenytoin (10 to 20 μG/ml) are being sought, but these signs generally disappear with reduction in dosage to provide plasma levels below 20 μG/ml. Occasionally phenytoin overdosage produces atypical neurological manifestations e.g. dyskinesia.

2. Effects on folic acid-vitamin B_{12} metabolism. Megaloblastic anaemia may occur in patients receiving phenytoin, primidone and, very rarely, phenobarbitone. When taken over a period of some years, these drugs may interfere with folic acid metabolism to such an extent that this produces megaloblastic anaemia. Examination of the peripheral blood may not clearly indicate folic acid disturbance and the diagnosis is best made by biopsy and examination of the bone marrow, or by estimating the serum folate level, which is generally below the normal lower limit of 5 picogram/ml. In such instances, folic acid should be given orally in addition to anticonvulsant therapy. However until more is known of the action of anticonvulsants, folic acid should not be given prophylactically to patients whose epilepsy is

satisfactorily controlled and who show no evidence of anaemia or folic acid deficiency.

Neuropsychiatric symptoms (e.g., depression, dementia, schizophrenic-like psychosis, peripheral neuropathy) may occur rarely in persons taking phenytoin over a number of years. Serum folate levels are low and serum vitamin B_{12} levels may be low or normal. Improvement in the patient's mental state may occur when vitamin B_{12} is given with folic acid. However, since plasma phenytoin levels fall when folic acid is given it is difficult to be sure of the mechanism of the symptoms.

3. Low serum protein-bound iodine. This finding in a patient with epilepsy receiving phenytoin might suggest an erroneous diagnosis of myxoedema. However, phenytoin does not cause subthyroidism and the low serum protein-bound iodine value is probably due to the drug interfering with the binding of thyroxine by plasma protein.

4. Hypocalcaemia. Prolonged anticonvulsant therapy with phenytoin, phenobarbitone or primidone may be associated with a fall in serum calcium concentration, and raised alkaline phosphatase levels. Occasionally osteomalacia has occurred. It is believed that the anticonvulsants accelerate the metabolism of vitamin D to biologically inactive products and so produce a relative deficiency state of biologically active vitamin D.

5. Immunological abnormalities. Various immunological abnormalities (e.g., low levels of IgA) have been reported with some frequency in patients taking phenytoin.

Effects on the foetus and neonate. The increased risk of developmental defects in the foetus associated with maternal phenytoin intake during pregnancy has already been mentioned. Babies born to mothers who have taken anticonvulsants during late pregnancy may have a deficiency in vitamin K dependent clotting factors at birth.

Suggested usage
At the present time phenytoin is probably the drug of first choice in all varieties of partial epilepsy (particularly those in which the seizures become secondarily generalised), and possibly major seizures of primary generalised epilepsy. It is of doubtful value in myoclonic seizures and febrile convulsions and has no direct value in petit mal absences. However, because specific therapy for petit mal epilepsy occasionally precipitates major seizures, phenytoin is often combined with a drug of the succinimide (e.g. ethosuximide) or oxazolidinedione group (e.g. troxidone) in treating petit mal absences. For other types of epilepsy, phenytoin may be combined with phenobarbitone, primidone, carbamazepine (Tegretol) or, particularly in the cortical seizures

of partial epilepsy, sulthiame (Ospolot), if phenytoin alone proves inadequate.

Phenytoin may be given intravenously to control status epilepticus (p. 133).

Preparations

Capsules or tablets; 30 mg, 50 mg and 100 mg.

Suspension; 30 mg in 5 ml and 100 mg in 5 ml.

Ampoules for parenteral use; 250 mg.

Average dosage

Under 1 year of age: 20 mg two or three times daily.
Under 6 years: 30 mg-100 mg twice daily.
Over 6 years: 60 mg-200 mg twice daily.

It has been found that initial phenytoin doses of 4–5 mg/kg body weight/day run very little risk of producing over-dosage side effects. If plasma phenytoin levels are measured one to two weeks after commencing this dosage the dose can subsequently be adjusted to produce plasma phenytoin levels in the desirable range of 10–20 μG/ml, bearing in mind the non-linear shape of the relation between plasma phenytoin level and phenytoin dose in the individual patient (Fig. 32). On a body weight basis, children under 12 need almost twice as much phenytoin as adults. If a rapid anticonvulsant effect is desired, a single oral loading dose of twice the expected daily maintenance dose may be given, with the maintenance dosage commencing 12 hours later.

Methoin (mephenytoin: Mesontoin: Mesantoin)

Methoin differs from phenytoin in two respects. Methoin has greater sedative properties, and a product of demethylation of methoin (Nirvanol), although an anticonvulsant, tends to be toxic to the bone marrow. Therefore, although methoin may sometimes be a more powerful anticonvulsant than phenytoin, its increased efficacy is offset by its increased toxicity rendering it much less suitable for routine use. Serious toxic effects of blood dyscrasias and liver damage, in addition to other side effects of the hydantoin group, may be encountered in a considerable proportion of cases treated with the drug. The use of methoin should be restricted to the situation where all other appropriate anticonvulsants have failed. The peripheral blood picture should be monitored with great care if the drug must be used.

Preparations
Tablets; 100 mg

Average dosage
Under 1 year of age: 25 mg twice daily.
Under 6 years: 25–50 mg twice to three times daily.
Over 6 years: 50–100 mg three to four times daily.

Ethotoin (Peganone)

Although ethotoin is of low toxicity, it has a relatively low potency. The drug can be employed in grand mal epilepsy if side effects of phenytoin and other appropriate anticonvulsants prove prohibitive.

Preparations
Tablets; 250 mg and 500 mg.

Average dosage
Under 1 year of age: 125 mg two to three times daily.
Under 6 years: 125–250 mg three times daily.
Over 6 years: 250–500 mg three to four times daily.

DIBENZAZEPINE DERIVATIVES

Carbamazepine (Tegretol)
Carbamazepine is a dibenzazepine derivative and is thus chemically related to the tricyclic antidepressant imipramine (Tofranil). Carbamazepine has the structural formula:

This drug now has an established place in the treatment of tic douloureux (trigeminal neuralgia) and also has potent anticonvulsant properties, being particularly effective in controlling major tonic-clonic seizures and focal cortical seizures. It has little or no effect on petit mal. Its alleged psychotropic effect may be of some advantage in the treatment of emotionally disturbed epileptic children. Carbamazepine can be given in combination with phenytoin, phenobarbitone or primidone. Carbamazepine appears to have established itself as a major first-line anticonvulsant. In its pharmacological properties it is probably more similar to phenytoin than to any other anticonvulsant. Because it does not produce hirsutism, it may be preferred in treating younger females.

Side effects
Although generally well tolerated, carbamazepine may produce side effects: 'allergic' skin reactions, drowsiness, dry mouth and gastrointestinal disturbance. Jaundice has been reported and fatal aplastic anaemia has occurred rarely. The drug has sedative properties and in overdosage can cause drowsiness and ataxia. It may cause water retention and, rarely, water intoxication. Although no teratogenic effect has been reported on the human foetus, there is some evidence of teratogenicity in laboratory animals and it is probably preferable to avoid introducing carbamazepine during the first three months of pregnancy in a patient with epilepsy.

Suggested usage
In addition to its value in controlling trigeminal neuralgia, carbamazepine can be given to control grand mal generalised epilepsy and all patterns of partial seizure. The possible psychotropic effect of the drug can be taken advantage of in children with temporal lobe seizures associated with disturbed behaviour. The drug may be of some use in milder forms of myoclonic generalised epilepsy. The therapeutic range of plasma carbamazepine level appears to be $6-12 \mu G/ml$. However the drug forms an epoxide metabolite which is also an anticonvulsant in experimental animals. The correlations between plasma carbamazepine-epoxide levels and anticonvulsant effect in man are not known. When phenytoin is used in conjunction with carbamazepine, plasma carbamazepine levels fall appreciably but carbamazepine-epoxide levels are largely unaltered. It is therefore possible that the therapeutic ranges of plasma carbamazepine level may be lower in the presence of phenytoin than in its absence, because of the equal contribution of carbamazepine-epoxide to the anticonvulsant effect in both circumstances.

There is so little correlation between steady-state plasma carbamazepine level and oral carbamazepine dose that only rough guidelines to appropriate carbamazepine dose can be offered, as below. Plasma level monitoring is needed to determine the potential adequacy of the dose.

Preparations
Tablets; 200 mg

Average dosage
Under 1 year of age: 50–100 mg twice daily.
Under 6 years: 100 mg two or three times daily.
Over 6 years: 100–200 mg two to four times daily.

BARBITURATE ANTICONVULSANTS

Phenobarbitone was the first effective organic anticonvulsant. It and its congeners are relatively similar in structure, and the barbiturates

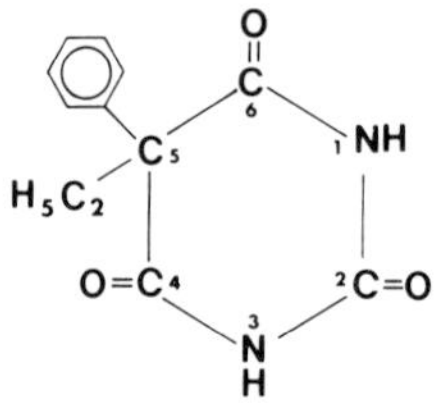

Phenobarbitone

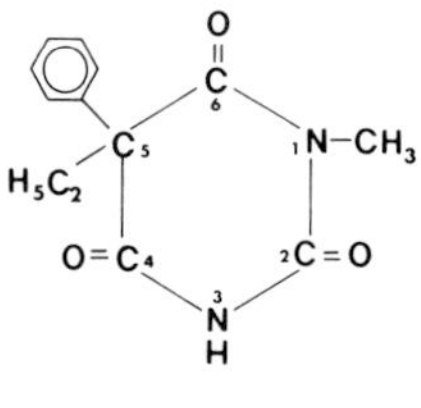

Methylphenobarbitone

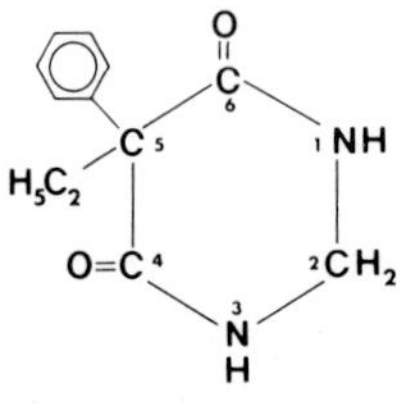

Primidone

also resemble the hydantoins in structure except that there is an additional carbon atom in the barbiturate ring.

The structures of primidone and phenobarbitone are identical except that the carbonyl group at the C_2 position of phenobarbitone is reduced to a CH_2 group in primidone. Although methylphenobarbitone has an anticonvulsant action it is demethylated by the liver, while primidone (also an anticonvulsant in its own right) is oxidised by the liver. Thus both drugs are biotransformed to phenobarbitone. Therefore it might be argued that both methylphenobarbitone and primidone are largely, though not entirely, pro-drugs for phenobarbitone, and it would be simpler, and cheaper, to prescribe the latter directly. However primidone has achieved a widespread use in its own right, while methylphenobarbitone has the peculiar advantage that steady-state plasma phenobarbitone levels derived from it rise in direct proportion to methylphenobarbitone dose, whereas steady-state plasma phenobarbitone levels rise in a non-linear fashion when phenobarbitone itself is prescribed.

Phenobarbitone
Phenobarbitone is a potent anticonvulsant and is also cheap and safe. It is of value in controlling all varieties of partial epilepsy, tonic-clonic seizures of generalised epilepsy, febrile convulsions and sometimes myoclonic seizures. It acts as a depressant of both the cortex and the reticular formation in the brain stem.

Side effects
1. In effective anticonvulsant dosage, phenobarbitone tends to produce sedation.
2. In children, the drug not infrequently produces irritability and restlessness.
3. Psychic manifestations of temporal lobe epilepsy may be aggravated.
4. Ataxia may be produced.
5. Occasionally a rash develops.
6. The possible effects of phenobarbitone on calcium metabolism, foetal development and blood coagulation in the neonate have already been mentioned.

Suggested usage
To treat grand mal epilepsy whether of primarily or secondarily generalised origin, febrile convulsions of infancy and all varieties of partial epilepsy. Phenobarbitone may be combined with phenytoin, carbamazepine, ethosuximide or the newer anticonvulsants. It is not

rational to combine it with methylphenobarbitone or primidone since this is equivalent to giving more phenobarbitone. For most forms of epilepsy the therapeutic range of plasma phenobarbitone level appears to be 10–30 μG/ml (15–30 μG/ml for febrile convulsions).

Preparations
Tablets: 15 mg, 30 mg, 60 mg, 100 mg.
Elixir: 5 mg per ml.

Average dosage
Under 1 year of age: 15 mg once or twice daily.
Under 6 years: 30 mg once or twice daily.
Over 6 years: 60–100 mg once or twice daily.

Methylphenobarbitone (Prominal)
Methylphenobarbitone has the same spectrum of anti-epilepsy action and the same pattern of adverse effects as phenobarbitone. Under steady-state conditions plasma methylphenobarbitone levels are about 1/7th to 1/10th of the simultaneous plasma phenobarbitone levels, so that the greater part of the anticonvulsant effect of methylphenobarbitone almost certainly derives from the phenobarbitone formed from it. Plasma phenobarbitone levels form an adequate guide to methylphenobarbitone therapy. The two drugs can be used interchangably, but it should be remembered that 1 mg of phenobarbitone will yield the same plasma phenobarbitone level as nearly 2 mg of methylphenobarbitone. The reason for this discrepancy in dosage is not known, though it is probably not poor absorption of methylphenobarbitone. If the difference in dosage of the two drugs is forgotten patients can easily become overdosed when their treatment is changed from methylphenobarbitone to phenobarbitone, or underdosed if changed from phenobarbitone to methylphenobarbitone.

Preparations
Tablets: 30, 60 and 200 mg

Dosage
Under 1 year of age: 30 mg once or twice daily.
Under 6 years: 30–60 mg once or twice daily.
Over 6 years: 60–200 mg once or twice daily.

Primidone (Mysoline)
Primidone may be effective in patients with tonic-clonic seizures of primarily or secondarily generalised type, myoclonic seizures and all

varieties of partial epilepsy. The drug has not yet been proven superior to phenobarbitone when both drugs are given in doses that produce similar plasma phenobarbitone levels.

Side effects

1. The principal drawback to primidone therapy is the tendency of the drug to cause hypersomnia. This is particularly noticeable at the beginning of therapy and for this reason the drug should be introduced in very low dosage which is gradually increased over a few weeks.
2. A syndrome of vertigo and ataxia, sometimes with diplopia, may occur during the first few days of treatment.
3. Occasionally, a rash develops.
4. Primidone may cause megaloblastic anaemia and possibly leucopenia.
5. Although the drug can be used in partial epilepsy, there is a tendency for psychotic reactions to be precipitated by primidone in patients suffering from temporal lobe epilepsy and for this reason it has been suggested that it is better to avoid a combination of primidone (Mysoline) and sulthiame (Ospolot).

Suggested usage

1. Primidone is of value in tonic-clonic seizures either primarily or secondarily generalised in nature, either alone or in combination with phenytoin. It is irrational to combine primidone and phenobarbitone.
2. Primidone is of value in myoclonic epilepsy, and all varieties of partial epilepsy.

Primidone itself has a relatively short half-life in plasma and plasma levels of the drug can show considerable variation across a dosage interval. Therefore, although therapeutic ranges for plasma primidone levels have been quoted, it is probably more satisfactory to use plasma phenobarbitone levels as a guide to primidone therapy.

Preparations
Tablets: 50 mg, 250 mg.
Suspension: 25 mg per ml.

Dosage
Under 1 year of age: 50 mg twice to four times daily.
Under 6 years: 50–100 mg twice to four times daily.
Over 6 years: 100–250 mg twice to four times daily.

Primidone dosage should be adjusted to produce plasma pheno-barbitone level of 10 to 25 μG/ml, unless lower doses prove effective.

SUCCINIMIDE DERIVATIVES

The succinimide drugs were developed in an attempt to obtain a drug effective against petit mal, yet with minimal adverse effects. Three preparations are available: phensuximide (Milontin), methsuximide (Celontin) and ethosuximide (Zarontin).

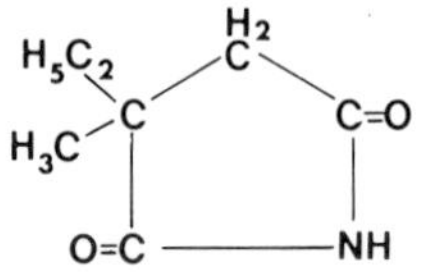

Ethosuximide

All three drugs are useful in the control of petit mal. However ethosuximide (Zarontin) is the most effective, being regarded by many neurologists as the drug of first choice in this condition. Ethosuximide has, however, a tendency to evoke major convulsive seizures in patients with petit mal attacks. When it is used the patient should also be given a drug effective in controlling grand mal to counteract this tendency. Phensuximide (Milontin) has less tendency to evoke major seizures but is less effective therapeutically. Methsuximide (Celontin) is more potent than phensuximide; there is no evidence that major seizures may be occasioned by this drug and, indeed, methsuximide is occasionally useful in the treatment of partial (cortical) seizures.

Side effects
In addition to some tendency for ethosuximide (Zarontin) to evoke grand mal attacks, side effects common to the succinimide group of drugs include gastrointestinal upset (anorexia, nausea, vomiting), an 'allergic' rash, lethargy (sometimes amounting to a dream-like state), pancytopenia and leucopenia.

Suggested usage

1. The control of petit mal absence epilepsy.
2. Methsuximide (Celontin) is occasionally helpful in controlling partial, (symptomatic, cortical) epilepsy and can be given with phenytoin for this purpose.
3. Ethosuximide has some action against myoclonic seizures of generalised epilepsy.

Preparations
Phensuximide capsules, 500 mg.
Methsuximide capsules, 300 mg.
Ethosuximide capsules, 250 mg.
Ethosuximide syrup, 250 mg in 5 ml.

Average dosage
Under 6 years of age: phensuximide or methsuximide, one or two capsules per day; ethosuximide, 250 mg to 750 mg daily. Over 6 years of age: phensuximide or methsuximide, one capsule per day for first week. If required, dosage is increased by one capsule each week to a maximum of four capsules daily. Ethosuximide, one capsule (250 mg) daily for first week. Second week, two capsules daily. If necessary, the dose can be increased by one capsule per week until side effects occur or the petit mal absences are controlled. The therapeutic range of plasma ethosuximide level appears to be 40–120 μG/ml. However plasma ethosuximide level monitoring is rarely necessary as an aid to therapy since absence seizures occur frequently so that response to therapy can be readily determined on clinical grounds. The ability to measure plasma ethosuximide levels may help check that the patients are complying with their prescribed dosage regimes.

BENZODIAZEPINE DERIVATIVES

Several benzodiazepine derivatives possess anticonvulsant activity. Those in current use are diazepam (Valium), nitrazepam (Mogadon), and clonazepam (Rivotril; Clonopin). The structural formulae of these drugs are shown below:

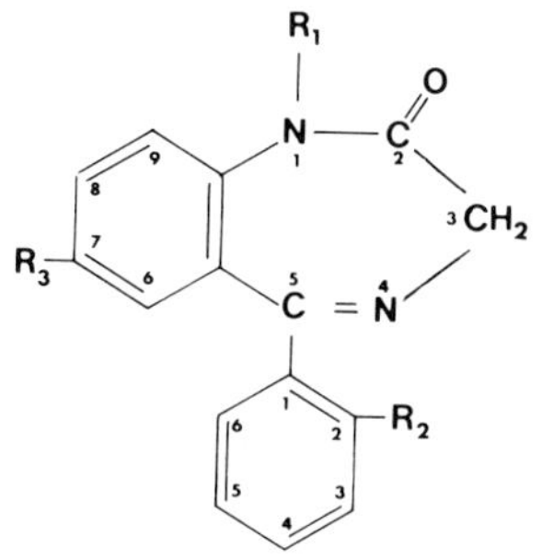

	R$_1$	R$_2$	R$_3$
Diazepam	$-CH_3$	$-H$	$-Cl$
Nitrazepam	$-H$	$-H$	$-NO_2$
Clonazepam	$-H$	$-Cl$	$-NO_2$

Other derivatives e.g. lorazepam, are currently being investigated.

In general, this group of drugs raises the after-discharge threshold of the thalamus but not the cortex, in this respect resembling troxidone rather than phenobarbitone and phenytoin (these drugs tend to raise the threshold of both thalamus and cortex). Diazepam and especially nitrazepam increase the after-discharge threshold of the amygdala.

Side effects
These are not particularly troublesome but some patients complain of sedation, fatigue, muscle hypotonus or ataxia. Clonazepam sometimes appears to cause irritability and aggressiveness.

Suggested usage
Diazepam appears to be finding its main role as an anticonvulsant when given parenterally to control status epilepticus. Nitrazepam, given orally, is often an effective drug for myoclonic varieties of generalised epilepsy, while clonazepam has perhaps the broadest spectrum of antiepilepsy action of the anticonvulsants currently available. Parenterally it is an effective agent for status epilepticus. Orally it is often efficacious for both absence and myoclonic seizures of generalised epilepsy; it is useful for tonic-clonic seizures of generalised epilepsy, and sometimes is helpful in controlling partial epilepsy, particularly when the seizures originate in a temporal lobe.

Preparations
Diazepam: tablets   2mg, 5mg and 10mg.
              syrup   2mg in 5ml.
              ampoules 10mg.
Nitrazepam: tablets   5mg.
Clonazepam: tablets   0.5mg, 2mg.
              ampoules 1mg.

Average dosage
Diazepam: 5-20mg parenterally, as necessary.
Nitrazepam: 5-20mg per day.
Clonazepam: 0.5mg twice daily to 4mg twice daily.

Although it is possible to monitor plasma concentrations of the benzodiazepine anticonvulsants therapeutic ranges for the various drugs have not been established and the plasma level data are of little use clinically.

VALPROIC ACID DERIVATIVES

Sodium valproate (sodium di-n-propyl acetate; sodium propyl-n-pentanoate; Epilim or Depakene) is the sodium salt of a branched chain fatty acid. Its anticonvulsant properties were discovered accidentally while it was being used as a solvent for other drugs. Sodium valproate has the following structural formula:

$$CH_3.CH_2.CH_2$$
$$CH.COOH$$
$$CH_3.CH_2.CH_2$$

The drug acts biochemically as an inhibitor of enzymes which metabolise the inhibitory synaptic transmitter gamma aminobutyric acid (GABA). It is thought that raised brain GABA levels produced by the drug have an antiepileptic effect.

Side effects
Sodium valproate may cause some gastrointestinal disturbance and, given in overdosage, weakness and ataxia, though relatively little sedation. There have been reports that it may cause a bleeding tendency and liver damage. Apparently animal studies have suggested that the drug, given in high dosage, may lead to testicular damage.

Suggested usage
Oral sodium valproate appears a very effective drug for generalised epilepsy of all types, but particularly for absence and myoclonic seizures. Its effectiveness in partial epilepsy is less clear as it has often been prescribed in conjunction with other anticonvulsants. Addition of valproate can cause a major rise in plasma phenobarbitone levels and changes in phenytoin levels, and these changes in concentration of other anticonvulsants make it difficult to determine the direct antiepileptic effect of valproate.

Preparations
Sodium valproate: tablets of 200 mg and 500 mg in individual foil wrapping (the drug is quite hygroscopic).

Average dosage
Under 6 years: Sodium valproate 100–200 mg three times a day.
Over 6 years: Sodium valproate 200–400 mg three or four times a day.
    The therapeutic range of plasma valproate level has been tentatively set at 50 to 100 μG/ml. Valproate has a comparatively short half-life in

plasma and, unlike most other anticonvulsants, its plasma levels may show considerable variation over a six to eight hour dosage interval.

MISCELLANEOUS MINOR ANTICONVULSANTS

Sulthiame (Ospolot)

Sulthiame is a butane sultam compound, structurally related to the sulphonamides:

$$\text{structure of sulthiame: butane-sultam ring} - \text{C}_6\text{H}_4 - \text{S(=O)}_2 - \text{NH}_2$$

The free $SO_2\text{-}NH_2$ group might suggest a carbonic anhydrase inhibiting effect similar to acetazolamide but the principal anti-convulsant activity of the molecule appears to be related to the butane-sultam ring.

The main indication for sulthiame would appear to be in the control of partial (cortical) epilepsy. For a number of years sulthiame has been used in conjunction with phenytoin. Evidence has now accumulated that sulthiame causes plasma phenytoin levels to rise, so that benefit apparently due to a direct antiepilepsy effect of sulthiame may really be due to a pharmacokinetic interaction that increased the anti-convulsant effect of phenytoin. The place of sulthiame as an anticonvulsant in its own right has now become rather uncertain.

Side effects

The most important limiting factor in sulthiame therapy is the occurrence of side effects. Although in many instances these symptoms subside within a week or two, in some 10 per cent of patients they are sufficiently troublesome to warrant discontinuance of the drug. These side effects include gastrointestinal upset, headache, hyperventilation, paraesthesiae, drowsiness and mental confusion.

There has also been some evidence that sulthiame may occasion status epilepticus but this seems to be related to the withdrawal of other anticonvulsants and we have not encountered this complication when sulthiame is added to phenytoin to obtain added anticonvulsant activity. It is not advised that sulthiame be used with primidone in the treatment of cortical (temporal lobe) epilepsy since it would appear that this combination may produce psychic side effects. When used in therapeutic dosage sulthiame does not seem to have any toxic effect on bone marrow or kidneys.

Suggested usage
In combination with phenytoin in the control of partial (cortical) epileptic seizures.

Preparations
Tablets of 50 mg and 200 mg.

Average dosage
Under 1 year of age: 50 mg daily or twice daily.
Under 6 years: 50–100 mg daily to three times daily.
Over 6 years: 100–200 mg twice to three times daily.

Acetazolamide (Diamox)

Acetazolamide is a sulphonamide derivative with pronounced anticarbonic anhydrase activity which appears to be related to the presence of an unsubstituted SO_2-NH_2 group:

$$CH_3-CO-NH-C\underset{S}{\overset{N-N}{\diagdown\diagup}}C-SO_2NH_2$$

It had been noticed previously that Prontosil and sulphanilamide had a tendency to reduce epileptic seizures whereas later sulphonamides (resulting from substitution on the free SO_2-NH_2 group) had no such activity. This anticonvulsant property appears to be related to the ability of acetazolamide to inhibit the enzyme carbonic anhydrase which catalyses the reversible reaction.

$$H_2O + CO_2 \rightleftharpoons H_2CO_3$$

Acetazolamide was found to have several hundred times the anticarbonic anhydrase activity of sulphanilamide and its mode of action in epilepsy may depend on direct inhibition of carbonic anhydrase which occurs in the nervous system of man, particularly in the thalamus. Acetazolamide may increase the intraneuronal concentration of CO_2 and diminish pH, thus simulating the inhibition of petit mal absence attacks by the inhalation of CO_2 (the converse to the precipitation of petit mal by hyperventilation which increases the excretion of CO_2 from the lungs, blood and brain). This would accord with the finding that acetazolamide is of most value as an adjuvant to other drugs in the control of petit mal absences, particularly when hyperventilation causes activation of seizures.

Side effects
These are uncommon but gastrointestinal disturbance, flushes, headache, fatigue and paraesthesiae have been encountered. There is some slight risk of calculus formation and renal colic.

Suggested usage
In patients suffering from petit mal epilepsy, as an adjuvant to succinimide or oxazolidineadione therapy, when the attacks are not satisfactorily controlled by these drugs alone and the newer anti-convulsants clonazepam and sodium valproate are unavailable, or cannot be used for some reason or other.

Preparations
Tablets; 250 mg.

Average dosage
Under 1 year of age: 125 mg daily or twice daily.
Under 6 years: 125–250 mg daily or twice daily.
Over 6 years: 250 mg daily to three times daily.

THE OXAZOLIDINEDIONES

These drugs were the first specific agents available for petit mal absence epilepsy. They are now largely superseded by more effective and less toxic drugs.

Troxidone (Tridione) and paramethadione (Paradione)
These two drugs are representative of the group; their structural formulae are very similar.

	R_1	R_2	R_3
Trimethadione	CH_3	CH_3	CH_3
Dimethadione	CH_3	CH_3	H
Paramethadione	CH_3	C_2H_5	CH_3

As might be expected, both drugs are also similar in therapeutic usage and dosage. Both control the epileptic manifestations and tend to normalise the electroencephalogram in many children suffering from petit mal absences.

Side effects
These are also similar and include sedation, glare phenomena (photophobia), skin rashes, tendency to evoke major seizures, neutropenia, aplastic anaemia and nephrosis.

On the whole paramethadione appears to have less tendency to produce side effects or toxic effects. In particular there is less tendency to evoke major seizures and 'glare' phenomena. Of more importance is the fact that if toxic symptoms develop to one of these drugs, it does not necessarily mean that the patient will be similarly affected by the other preparation.

In patients with petit mal absences it is often advisable to minimise the risk of major seizures occurring by prescribing a drug effective against major epilepsy in addition to troxidone or paramethadione. If such a drug combination is indicated, phenytoin (Dilantin) would seem to be the drug of choice particularly in view of the relative lack of sedation associated with this therapy. If it proves unsuitable phenobarbitone, primidone or carbamazepine could be substituted. Methoin should not be used with the oxazolidinediones because the combined toxic effects on the bone marrow may have serious consequences.

Suggested usage
The control of the petit mal absence type of generalised epilepsy.

Preparations
Troxidone tablets; 150 mg.
Troxidone capsules; 300 mg.
Paramethadione capsules; 300 mg.

Average dosage
Under 6 years: 150–300 mg three to four times daily.
Over 6 years: 300–600 mg three to four times daily.
Dosage is adjusted on clinical grounds to control petit mal absences.

Adrenocorticotropic hormone (and tetracosactrin)
Adrenocorticotropic hormone (ACTH) has been shown to be of value in the treatment of infantile spasms (hypsarrhythmia) particularly when there is no associated gross brain damage. In some instances, the clinical and electroencephalographic improvement may be dramatic, the seizures ceasing and a normal E.E.G. pattern being restored within two to three weeks. In other patients, although the hypsarrhythmic character of the E.E.G. may be lost, the tracing may remain abnormal and show evidence of focal or epileptic abnormalities. Even if ACTH

stops the myoclonic seizures of hypsarrhythmia, unless the patient has been treated within a few weeks of the onset of attacks it is unlikely that intellectural function will recover fully. The nature of the ACTH effect is not understood.

Suggested usage
Infantile spasms (hypsarrhythmia).

Preparations
Ampoules:
ACTH retard; Tetracosactrin.

Average dosage
An intramuscular injection of 25 international units of ACTH or 0.5–1 mg tetracosactrin depot daily. If the seizures are not improved or if the E.E.G. remains unchanged the dose should be increased to 50 i.u. of ACTH or 1–2 mg tetracosactrin daily for three or four weeks and continued thereafter in gradually decreasing doses for several months.

Routine anticonvulsants, such as phenytoin, can be given in addition.

Pyridoxine
Pyridoxine (vitamin B_6) has the structural formula:

Pyridoxine is concerned in the synthesis of at least one chemical inhibitory synaptic transmitter in the brain (gamma-amino-butyric acid) and certain animals and humans may develop convulsions if given a pyridoxine deficient diet. Clinically, a small number of infants presenting with infantile spasms has an alteration in tryptophan metabolism. These children require additional pyridoxine and a dramatic clinical response may follow administration of the vitamin.

No supplementary vitamin B_6 is given over a period of some 72 hours and then pyridoxine (1 mg per kg body weight) is administered intravenously. Clinical improvement and corresponding E.E.G. improvement occur within a short time thus indicates the nature of the underlying defect. Maintenance therapy (approximately 14 mg per kg body weight) can then be instituted orally.

Suggested usage
Certain patients with infantile spasms.

Preparations
Tablets;   10 mg, 25 mg, 50 mg.
Ampoules;   50 mg in 1 ml.

KETOGENIC DIET AND EPILEPSY

Before anticonvulsants were readily available for clinical use, some improvement in seizure control was possibly obtained by starvation for at least 48 hours or so until ketosis was induced. Workers at the Mayo Clinic then developed a high fat diet which also produced ketosis and this was shown to be effective in some cases in producing seizure control. The basic diet provides approximately 80 per cent of caloric requirements from fat, with protein and carbohydrate providing the remainder equally.

In the 50 odd years since its introduction, the popularity of this mode of treatment has waxed and waned. During this interval, many explanations of its mode of action have been proposed but still no satisfactory explanation is known. It is certainly not the ketosis alone which is effective and electrolyte imbalance, amino-acid fluxes, and increased serum lipids also have failed to provide the answer.

The indications for its use at present would seem to be in childhood epilepsy resistant to control with usual anticonvulsants, and best results are obtained when a focal cause is not present. The diet can be made more palatable by supplying the dietary fat in the form of medium chain triglycerides. It is perhaps worth noting that valproic acid, a branched chain fatty acid, is most effective for those types of epilepsy in which a ketogenic diet was often formerly used.

THE TECHNIQUE OF ANTICONVULSANT DRUG THERAPY

Table 9 indicates drugs of value in the various types of epilepsy. Having considered the history, the results of electroencephalography and any other relevant ancillary investigations, choose the safest, effective, appropriate anticonvulsant. Introduce the drug in a dose a little less than the mean dose suggested in Table 8. Thereafter make gradual dose increments generally not more often than once a week (to let tissue levels stabilise between dose changes) until control is achieved (or therapeutic blood levels are reached, if facilities for estimation of these exist), or until toxic effects appear.

If the seizures are controlled, continue with therapy for a period of at least three years.

If seizures are partially controlled by the first drug taken to its limit of tolerance, add the next safest effective preparation in gradually increasing doses.

If the first drug has no therapeutic effect or if unacceptable toxic effects appear, add the second safest effective anticonvulsant and gradually withdraw the first drug, continuing in this manner until an effective drug combination for each particular patient is found.

Maintenance therapy should be continued in full dosage to maintain total control of seizures for three to five years. During this protracted course of anticonvulsant therapy it is wise to keep the patient under observation every few months, both to provide psychological support and advice as to problems which arise, to encourage the patient to persist with the therapy and to comply with the prescribed dosages. Monitoring plasma drug levels at intervals helps ensure compliance. Such careful follow-up improves the prospects of long-term cure of epilepsy.

PLASMA ANTICONVULSANT LEVEL MONITORING

At various stages in the present chapter reference has been made to the monitoring of plasma anticonvulsant drug levels. This topic is one of growing importance and warrants some brief comment.

Monitoring plasma anticonvulsant levels may help the clinician in several ways:

1. It permits him to judge whether the prescribed dose of an anticonvulsant is likely to prove adequate long before the patient's clinical response indicates whether or not this is so.
2. It permits him to detect whether the patients' symptoms are likely to be due to overdosage.
3. It permits him to detect failures of patient compliance.
4. It permits him to detect pharmacokinetic interactions which might lead to symptoms or treatment failure that could be difficult to interpret clinically.

For optimal use to be made of the measurements the clinician should ensure that the appropriate substance is measured. Thus it is more helpful to know the plasma phenobarbitone level than the plasma primidone level in a patient given the latter drug. Measurements should not be made till long enough from a dosage change to ensure the patient is in a steady state as regards the drug. For anticonvulsants with relatively short half-lives (valproate and primidone) minimal (i.e. immediately predosage) plasma levels should be measured. These levels vary in the steady state less than levels measured at any other stage in the dosage interval. *Above all, the plasma drug level should be used as a guide to the management of the clinical situation, and not regarded as the chief criterion of adequate therapy.* The aim of anticonvulsant therapy is the complete control of epilepsy without unwanted effects of therapy, and not the attaining of a particular plasma anticonvulsant concentration. Perfectly satisfactory anticonvulsant drug doses should never be changed merely because plasma anticonvulsant levels are 'too high' or 'too low'.

SUMMARY

1.

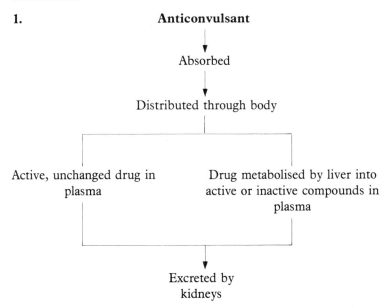

Anticonvulsant

Absorbed

Distributed through body

Active, unchanged drug in plasma

Drug metabolised by liver into active or inactive compounds in plasma

Excreted by kidneys

2. **Rate of metabolism of anticonvulsant** by liver may be variable due to genetic or acquired factors (other drugs, disease).

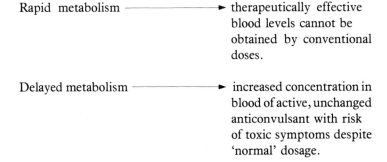

Rapid metabolism   ⟶   therapeutically effective blood levels cannot be obtained by conventional doses.

Delayed metabolism   ⟶   increased concentration in blood of active, unchanged anticonvulsant with risk of toxic symptoms despite 'normal' dosage.

3. The anticonvulsant drugs:

a. *Hydantoin* group ┬── phenytoin (Dilantin)
├── methoin (Mesantoin)
└── ethotoin (Peganone)

b. *Carbamazepine* (Tegretol)

c. *Barbiturates* ┬── phenobarbitone
├── methylphenobarbitone (Prominal)
└── primidone (Mysoline)

d. The *succinimides* ┬── phensuximide (Milontin)
├── methsuximide (Celontin)
└── ethosuximide (Zarontin)

e. *Benzodiazepines* ┬── diazepam (Valium)
├── nitrazepam (Mogadon)
└── clonazepam (Rivotril)

f. *Sodium valproate* (Epilim)

g. Miscellaneous minor anticonvulsants

   (i) sulthiame (Ospolot)
   (ii) acetazolamide (Diamox)
   (iii) the oxazolidinediones ┬── troxidone (Tridione)
   └── paramethadione (Paradione)
   (iv) adrenocorticotropic hormone (ACTH)
   (v) pyridoxine (vitamin B_6)

4. Anticonvulsants indicated for particular types of epilepsy

			First line drugs	Second line drugs
Generalised epilepsy		*Absences*	ethosuximide; clonazepam; valproate	troxidone
	Myoclonic Seizures			
	(i)	infantile	ACTH; tetracosactrin steroids	valproate
	(ii)	childhood	valproate: clonazepam	nitrazepam; ethosuximide; phenobarbitone
	(iii)	adolescence and later	valproate; clonazepam; phenobarbitone	carbamazepine
	Tonic-clonic Seizures		phenobarbitone; valproate	carbamazepine; phenytoin: clonazepam
Partial epilepsy	with or without secondary generalisation		phenytoin; phenobarbitone; carbamazepine	clonazepam; sulthiame; valproate; methoin

Note: Methylphenobarbitone or primidone can be substituted for phenobarbitone in the above.

5. The toxic effects of the commonly used anticonvulsants

Phenytoin (Dilantin)	Phenobarbitone	Primidone (Mysoline)
Gastric upset	Sedation	Sedation
Rash	Irritability	Vertigo, ataxia,
Gum hyperplasia		diplopia

Hirsutism	Ataxia	Megaloblastic anaemia
Nystagmus, ataxia	Rash	Leucopenia
Megaloblastic anaemia, (folate deficiency)	Foetal malformation	Precipitation of psychotic features
Leucopenia	Neonatal coagulation defect	
Lymphadenopathy	Hypocalcaemia	
Neuropsychiatric symptoms	Folate deficiency	
Hypocalcaemia		
Immunological abnormalities		
Foetal malformation (slight risk)		
Neonatal coagulation defect		

Methoin (Mesantoin)	**Carbamazepine** (Tegretol)	**Ethosuximide** (Zarontin)
as above + increased risk of liver damage and blood dyscrasia	Rash	May evoke major seizures
	Drowsiness	
	Gastrointestinal upset	Sedation,
	Jaundice	Lethargy
	Aplastic anaemia	Rash
	Water retention	Gastrointestinal upset
		Pancytopenia, Leucopenia

Sodium valproate (Epilim)	**Sulthiame** (Ospolot)	**Clonazepam** (Rivotril)
Gastrointestional upset	Gastrointestional upset	Drowsiness
Weakness	Paraesthesiae	Irritability and aggression
Ataxia	Headache	
Tremor	Drowsiness	
Bleeding tendency	Hyperventilation	
Liver damage		
?? Testicular atrophy	Mental confusion	

6. **Technique of anticonvulsant drug therapy**

  a. Consider history and electroencephalogram and choose the safest, effective, appropriate anticonvulsant.

  b. Gradually build up dosage until:
    (i) control achieved
    (ii) toxic effects occur
    (iii) therapeutic plasma levels achieved (if facilities available)

  c. If (i) seizures controlled—continue
    (ii) seizures partially controlled—continue in adequate dosage: add next safest, effective drug in gradually increasing dosage as in (b) above.
    (iii) seizures not influenced—add second safest effective drug and gradually withdraw first drug; depending on response continue as for (i) or (ii).

  d. When seizures controlled continue full anticonvulsant dosage for at least 3–5 years unless side effects indicate a dosage change.

7. **Information obtained from plasma anticonvulsant level monitoring**

  (i) potential adequacy of prescribed dose of anticonvulsants.
  (ii) whether overdosage has occurred.
  (iii) whether patient is taking the prescribed dosages.
  (iv) whether interactions are occurring when more than one drug is being taken.

FURTHER READING

Bochner F, Hooper W D, Tyrer J H, Eadie M J 1972 Effect of dosage increments on blood phenytoin concentrations. J Neurol Neurosurg Psychiat 35: 873
Eadie M J 1979 'Which anticonvulsant drug'. Drugs 17: 213
Eadie M J, Tyrer J H 1980 Anticonvulsant therapy. Pharmacological basis and practice. 2nd edn. Churchill Livingstone, Edinburgh
Eadie M J, Tyrer J H 1973 Plasma levels of anticonvulsants. Aust NZJ Med 3: 290
Loughnan P M, Gold H, Vance J C 1973 Phenytoin teratogenicity in man. Lancet 1: 70
Mann P, Eckert T, Tyrer J H, Sutherland J M 1967 Treatment of temporal lobe epilepsy with sulthiame (Ospolot): a follow-up study Med J Aust 2: 729
Reynolds E H, Preece J, Johnson A L 1971 Folate metabolism in epileptic and psychiatric patients. J Neurol Neurosurg Psychiat 34: 726
Richens A 1975 Drug treatment of epilepsy. Kimpton, London
Sparberg M 1963 Diagnostically confusing complications of diphenylhydantoin therapy. Ann Int Med 59: 914
Speidel B D, Meadow S R 1972 Maternal epilepsy and abnormalities of the fetus and new born. Lancet 2: 839
Stamp T C B, Round J M, Rowe D J F, Haddad J G 1972 Plasma levels and therapeutic effects of 25-hydroxycholecalciferol in epileptic patients taking anticonvulsant drugs. Brit Med J 4: 9

Wilson J 1969 Drug treatment of epilepsy in childhood. Brit Med J 2: 475
Woodbury D M, Penry J K, Schmidt R P 1972 Antiepileptic drugs. Raven Press, New York

8

Certain complications of epilepsy

The term status epilepticus embraces several different disturbances which are, however, all characterised by continuous epileptic activity.

1. Bilateral convulsive status.
2. Unilateral convulsive status.
3. Absence (Petit mal) status (in which almost continuous subclinical epileptic discharges may result in reversible mental deterioration).

Bilateral convulsive status epilepticus

The variety of status epilepticus which presents as a medical emergency is bilateral convulsive status. This is a condition in which one tonic-clonic epileptic seizure follows another without any intervening period of consciousness. This complication may occur in either generalised or partial epilepsy.

Bilateral convulsive status epilepticus may present in two ways:

1. *As the first manifestation of epilepsy*. This is not uncommon when the epileptogenic focus is in a frontal lobe. In such cases the status may prove very resistant to treatment. Because of this, hospital admission is generally desirable.

2. *As a complication in a patient with established epilepsy*. Under these circumstances, the development of status epilepticus may be preceded by an increased frequency of seizures. When repeated seizures occur each day but with recovery of consciousness between seizures, the condition can be described as *serial epilepsy* and should be regarded as a warning that bilateral convulsive status may be imminent. This may, however, be averted by intensive home therapy (routine anticonvulsants given in larger dosage and, perhaps, intravenously rather than orally at first). If seizures continue despite this, the patient should be admitted to hospital.

Convulsive status epilepticus occurring in a patient whose seizures have previously been controlled generally proves due either to omission of anticonvulsants or to the development of progressive brain disease.

Dangers

The dangers of bilateral convulsive status epilepticus include the following:

1. If convulsions continue coma deepens, pyrexia and hyperpyrexia may develop, signs of decompensation appear in the heart, lungs and kidneys, electrolyte imbalance may occur, and the patient may then die.
2. Even if the patient recovers from status epilepticus, permanent hypoxic neuronal damage leading to cerebral atrophy and dementia may have occurred.
3. Over-vigorous therapy with an anticonvulsant agent may result in cardiac or respiratory arrest or both.
4. Aspiration of secretions or vomitus may occur, leading to lung infection.

There is good evidence that the longer generalised convulsive status continues, the greater the mortality and morbidity. It is, therefore, necessary to have an effective therapeutic regime available and to commence it immediately.

Management

In the management of status epilepticus attention must be paid to the following:

1. Suppression of the seizures.
2. Institution of effective maintenance anticonvulsant therapy.
3. Maintenance of adequate airway and of fluid and electrolyte balance.
4. Diagnosis of the cause of the status and its remedy by appropriate measures if such are available.

Suppression of seizures

Diazepam (Valium) controls status epilepticus in the majority of instances, often within 2 to 10 minutes when the drug is given intravenously. Intramuscular injection is less efficient as the drug absorbs rather slowly.

Dosage. Diazepam (Valium) 1 to 2 mg per year of life to a maximum of 10 mg intravenously (or intramuscularly if intravenous injection is not practicable). This can be repeated if seizures recur, or 50 mg in 500 ml saline can be given by slow intravenous drip.

Clonazepam. Intravenous clonazepam (1–2 mg for adults and correspondingly less on a body weight basis for children) is probably a more effective agent than diazepam.

Phenytoin (Dilantin) 20 to 30 mg per year of life to a maximum of 250 mg (in children under 10 years of age to a maximum of 150 mg) may be given intravenously as a single dose. However, for an adult patient not already taking phenytoin, approximately 1 G must be given intravenously to obtain a 'therapeutic' level. This dose must be given intravenously over several hours. There is danger that the drug may precipitate out if it is injected into the fluid in a drip bottle, so that the patient may not receive the full dose intended. Therefore the parenteral solution of the drug is better injected at intervals into the tubing of an intravenous drip. The rate of infusion should not be so fast that hypotension occurs. Phenytoin absorbs so slowly from intra-muscular injection sites that this route of administration cannot be recommended.

In infants and very young children it is possible to give anticonvulsant drugs intravenously by utilising a scalp vein (Fig. 33).

Other drugs. Sodium phenobarbitone. Intramuscularly. For adults,

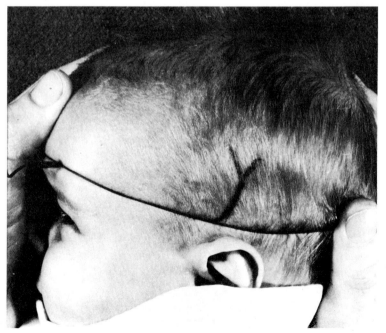

Fig. 33 Scalp vein.

200 mg; under one year of age, 50 mg; 1 to 4 years, 100 mg; 5 to 10 years, 120 mg.

Sodium amylobarbitone. A 5 per cent solution intravenously, 1 ml (i.e. 50 mg) per min until seizures cease or until a maximum of 10 ml has been administered. Watch for (i) respiratory depression and (ii) rapid fall in blood pressure.

Paraldehyde. Intramuscularly, or intravenously injected into a glucose saline or plasma drip. Under 1 year of age, 1 or 1.5 ml; up to 5 years, 3 ml; up to 10 years, 8 ml. Paraldehyde may dissolve the plastic in syringes or tubing.

Thiopentone. An initial intravenous dose of 25 to 100 mg is given slowly until convulsions cease; an intravenous drip is then set up (1 G in 500 ml of Ringer lactate solution) at a rate of 0.5 to 1 ml per min for 12 hours.

Chlormethiazole. An intravenous infusion of the 0.8 per cent solution is run at the rate of 4 ml per min till convulsing stops or undesirable effects occur.

Maintenance therapy

With the probable exception of phenobarbitone, the commonly used anticonvulsants that are available in solution appears to absorb more slowly after intramuscular than after oral administration. Therefore, unless phenobarbitone is to be used, it is often best to provide anticonvulsants intravenously till the patient can swallow. The drugs appropriate for maintenance use to prevent relapse of bilateral convulsive status are phenytoin, carbamazepine and phenobarbitone (or methylphenobarbitone, or primidone). If one of these drugs has been used to control the status, the maintenance dose initially should be a little greater than the usual expected maintenance dose of that drug. Later, the definitive dosage can be worked out. If the maintenance drug has not been used to control the status, a loading dose of twice the expected daily maintenance dose should be given, and maintenance dosage commenced 12 hours later.

Maintenance of airway and fluid-electrolyte balance

A clear airway must be maintained by (1) aspiration, (2) positioning, (3) inserting a simple airway and, if necessary, (4) performing tracheotomy and providing assisted respiration. Oxygen may be helpful in reducing cerebral anoxia and thus may help in controlling seizures.

Fluid balance must be carefully checked and serum electrolytes and blood urea estimated, at intervals, so that disturbances can be corrected.

Investigation of cause

If generalised convulsive status occurs as the first manifestation of epilepsy, a full neurological assessment is necessary once the seizures are controlled. Since such patients often prove to have a lesion in one or other frontal lobe, in addition to full clinical examination, X-rays of skull and chest, electroencephalography and C.T. scanning are often necessary, and other ancillary investigations (angiography or air studies) may be indicated.

On the other hand, status epilepticus may occur in a patient with established epilepsy who has previously been fully assessed. In such patients it is important to determine why status epilepticus should have occurred at this time. The most common explanation is that the patient has omitted to take the prescribed anticonvulsant drugs. This may be confirmed by questioning the patient when he regains consciousness. Blood should be taken for subsequent measurement of plasma anticonvulsant levels before drug therapy to control the status epilepticus is begun.

In rare instances, impaired absorption, overactive metabolism, or the effect of other drugs may be responsible for reduced effectiveness of anticonvulsants. Again, estimating the serum levels of the anticonvulsants (if a technique to do so is readily available) may prove useful. In still other patients, an intercurrent disease may act as a 'trigger' mechanism, or a previously treated condition, such as a meningioma, may have recurred and will necessitate reinvestigation and further treatment.

Unilateral convulsive status epilepticus

Focal motor status (epilepsia partialis continuans) occurs typically when a progressive pathology, encephalitic, vascular or neoplastic, involves one cerebral hemisphere. It may also occur in the presence of non-progressive unilateral pathology.

Clinically, unilateral status is characterised by repetitive myoclonic jerks involving the muscles of a limb or both limbs on one side, continuing in a regular or irregular manner for hours or days. The movements occur in the absence of any apparent stimulation and appear to be related to damage to inhibitory mechanisms in the cerebrum.

The most useful drug therapy appears to be clonazepam or diazepam which, initially, may have to be given parenterally to be effective. Phenobarbitone may be useful.

Absence status

This condition may be benign and reversible, or 'malignant' and due to progressive brain pathology.

Typically, benign absence status presents in childhood with *mental symptoms* (apathy, impaired concentration, deteriorating scholastic performance, confusion, changed behaviour) or *physical symptoms* (incoordination of hands, ataxic gait, myoclonic jerks), or a combination of both.

The *diagnosis* has to be differentiated from overdose of anticonvulsant drugs, folate acid deficiency due to these drugs, encephalopathy, posterior fossa tumour, and hydrocephalus due to aqueduct stenosis or fourth ventricle outlet stenosis.

The *electroencephalogram* shows virtually continuous generalised epileptic discharges often of 3 Hz or slower spike and wave type.

Rarely, a condition resembling absence status (epileptic pseudodementia) may occur when continuing localised epileptic discharges occur around a cortical focus situated some distance from the Rolandic area. The E.E.G. permits differentiation from absence status and anticonvulsants such as phenytoin or phenobarbitone may reverse the condition.

Treatment
In the typical benign case, complete recovery can be anticipated by employing adequate anticonvulsant drug therapy (ethosuximide, clonazepam or valproate).

EPILEPTIC PERSONALITY

It is very doubtful whether this exists as a true genetic trait. The combination of social rejection, institutionalisation and depressant effects of some anticonvulsants almost certainly accounts for many of the features of the so-called epileptic personality—slowness and rigidity of thinking and reaction, self-centredness, hypochondriasis and fixed opinions. Underlying brain pathology, resulting in some intellectual deficit as well as the epilepsy, accounts for other features. In general, the range of personality traits in patients suffering from epilepsy does not differ from that of the general population and particularly that section disadvantaged by chronic illnesses.

Episodes of irritability and aggressiveness with only minor or at times no provocation occur in some patients with so-called epileptic personalities, but last usually only minutes or hours. The question of whether or not these episodes are epileptic was mentioned in Chapter 3.

EPILEPTIC PSYCHOSES

Confusional states usually lasting hours occur in some patients with generalised epilepsy. These may occur following a seizure or be associated with a period of considerably disturbed and paroxysmal E.E.G. activity in the absence of overt seizures. Some of these instances merge into absence status.

Schizophrenic-like psychoses lasting days or weeks occur with a greater frequency in patients with temporal lobe epilepsy than in those with other forms. Behaviour may be grossly disturbed with paranoid thinking, hallucinations and serious homicidal or suicidal actions. These socially dangerous reactions, however, are rare. There is some evidence that these psychoses may be chronic in some patients, and in others they may be precipitated by drug therapy or drug-induced folate deficiency.

EPILEPTIC DETERIORATION

Apart from the chronic psychosis mentioned above, deterioration, both intellectual and social, occurs in some patients with very frequent seizures or recurrent status epilepticus. This deterioration in some, is almost certainly due to anoxic brain damage sustained in the seizures but in most is merely one further aspect of the underlying pathological process. Rarely it is due to unrecognised chronic anticonvulsant overdosage.

SUMMARY

1. Bilateral status epilepticus dangers

    a. Hyperpyrexia ⟶ deepening coma ⟶ death.
    b. Permanent neuronal damage.
    c. Aspiration of secretions and vomit.
    d. Therapy may lead to cardiac or respiratory arrest.

Management

    a. Suppress seizures ⸢ diazepam or clonazepam
                        ⸤ amylobarbitone; phenytoin
    b. Institute maintenance anticonvulsant therapy.
    c. Maintenance of airway and fluid-electrolyte balance.
    d. Determine and treat cause of status.

2. Unilateral status epilepticus

3. Absence status ⸢ Benign
                       ⸤ Malignant

4. Epileptic personality

Result of social rejection and
depressant effect of some
anticonvulsants

Underlying pathology

Intellectual   Epilepsy
deficit

Slowness and rigidity of thinking
Slow reactions
Self-centredness
Hypochondriasis

5. Epileptic psychosis ⎯ confusional states
 schizophrenia-like psychoses

6. Epileptic deterioration ⎯ intellectual
 social

Causes:
    (i) hypoxia during seizures
  (ii) progressive brain disease
 (iii) unrecognised anticonvulsant overdosage

FURTHER READING

Gastaut H, Naquet R, Poire R, Tassinari C A 1965 Treatment of status epilepticus
with diazepam (Valium). Epilepsia 6: 167
Gastaut H, Catier J, Dravet C, Roger J 1970 Exceptional anticonvulsive properties of
a new benzodiazepine. Epilepsy. Mod Probl Pharmacopsychiat 4: 261
Lalji D, Hosking C S, Sutherland J M 1967 Diazepam (Valium) in the control of
status epilepticus. Med J Aust 1: 542
Parsonage M J, Norris J W 1967 Use of diazepam in treatment of severe convulsive
status epilepticus. Brit Med J 3: 85
Wallis W, Kutt H, McDowell F 1968 Intravenous diphenylhydantoin in treatment of
acute repetitive seizures. Neurology (Minneap) 18: 513

9

The surgical treatment of epilepsy

It is not the purpose of this chapter to discuss neurosurgical techniques in relation to epilepsy but rather to indicate, in a general way, the type of patient suffering from epilepsy who might benefit from operative treatment. In only a very small proportion of patients is surgery indicated.

Generalised epilepsy
At the present time there is no acceptable surgical technique for the amelioration of primary generalised epilepsy of hereditary origin, or the vast majority of cases of acquired origin.

Partial (symptomatic) epilepsy
On the other hand, partial epilepsy may be caused by a condition which is susceptible to surgical treatment. Indeed, this is one reason why patients with partial epilepsy should be carefully assessed.

Extracranial causes
Epileptic seizures (partial, or rarely generalised) resulting from an extracranial cause, such as *hypoglycaemia*, often prove resistant to drug therapy. Control can only be achieved when the cause has been corrected e.g. when the islet cell adenoma in the pancreas has been surgically removed.

Intracranial causes
Intracranial lesions such as *meningioma* and *cerebral abscess* should be treated surgically in their own right. If epilepsy has occurred as a presenting symptom of these conditions, the seizures may continue post-operatively; however control by appropriate drug therapy is generally possible.

Surgical excision of a *post-traumatic cortical scar* is sometimes of value in reducing the tendency to seizures when adequate control by drug therapy has proved impossible. In such instances, the site of the cicatrix must be taken into consideration if the production of an important neurological deficit is to be avoided. Further, although the replacement of an area of glial, mesodermal and sometimes osteoid tissue by surgical cicatrix is rational and often beneficial no guarantee of success can be offered to the patient or his relatives.

Porencephalic cysts are often of congenital origin but may result from trauma. These cysts may communicate with the related ventricle by a narrow channel or may be simply an expansion of a portion of the ventricle. An epileptogenic focus or series of foci may be present in the wall of such cysts and surgical excision may prove a useful measure in helping to control the seizures when they have proved resistant to anticonvulsant drug therapy alone.

Arteriovenous malformations not infrequently present with epileptic seizures and as the thin walled veins of the malformation become increasingly varicose so may the surrounding cerebral cortex become increasingly epileptogenic. However, although haemorrhage from an arteriovenous malformation may indicate the desirability of neuro-surgery, the association of epilepsy with an arteriovenous malform-ation should not necessarily indicate surgery in preference to anticonvulsant drug therapy. Although haemorrhage is a potential risk, this complication of arteriovenous malformation is not invariable and the risk of producing a neurological deficit by surgery, particularly if the malformation is in the dominant hemisphere, must be weighed against the possible advantages of operation. A careful neurological-neurosurgical assessment of such patients is essential.

In some children with *cerebral palsy*, (particularly hemiparesis) associated with epilepsy and due to extensive atrophy of one cerebral hemisphere, the operation of hemispherectomy may help control seizures and improve behaviour. Although a formidable undertaking, and although these patients constitute a relatively small group, the operation is worth considering in children with intractable epilepsy (or gross behavioural disturbances) associated with hemiplegia, yet with good function in the remainder of the brain. The motor deficit may not be greatly increased and spasticity may even be lessened. In other patients with lesser degrees of cerebral palsy, yet with intractable seizures arising from the damaged hemisphere, lesser resections may result in improved seizure control.

An important group of patients is that in which *temporal lobe seizures* occur despite optimal anticonvulsant drug therapy, yet no structural abnormality can be detected clinically. In the first and second decades of life, incisural sclerosis (p. 25) is often responsible; in older patients, a small benign tumour such as a hamartoma, undetectable until operation, may be present. In such patients, the operation of temporal lobectomy may be considered (this consists of excision of the anterior and median part of one temporal lobe including the uncus, amygdala and hippocampus). This operation can be carried out on one side only since bilateral amputation of the temporal poles produces in man, as in monkeys, an affectless apathy, severe disturbance of memory and a tendency to uninhibited sexual activity. In the assessment of such patients, electroencephalography may clearly indicate a consistent unilateral focus. Unfortunately however, a unilateral lesion in one hemisphere may give rise to secondary abnormal electrical activity with epileptic characteristics on the opposite side. The clinician is then faced with the problems as to whether the patient has a bilateral lesion or whether the bilateral temporal spikes on the E.E.G. are due to a lesion on one side only with spread to the other, and, if so, which side is affected by the lesion. In such instances helpful information may be obtained from sphenoidal lead electroencephalography, particularly if the patient is given a barbiturate in sufficient dosage to produce drowsiness and light sleep. A diminution in one temporal lobe of the normal barbiturate-induced fast activity is useful evidence that this is the temporal lobe which is abnormal. C.T. scanning and air encephalography should also be employed in the assessment of such patients since these studies may indicate an abnormal dilation of one temporal horn. To complete the assessment an angiogram should be performed on the appropriate side (if this has not already been done) to exclude a vascular space occupying lesion such as a meningioma or arteriovenous malformation.

In such patients with temporal lobe epilepsy who have proved resistant to anticonvulsant drug therapy, anterior temporal lobectomy, preferably guided by cortical electroencephalography and cortical stimulation, may prove of value in reducing the tendency to seizures. Complications can occur—hemiparesis and visual field defects, and, if the dominant hemisphere is involved, dysphasia and auditory agnosia may result. The risks of complications must be weighed against the degree of disability experienced by the patient from his epilepsy. In general, one tends to restrict operative treatment on this group to patients who are hopelessly incapacitated by uncontrollable epileptic seizures or whose behavioural disorders associated with temporal lobe epilepsy necessitate institutional care. In certain instances lobotomy (the section of nerve fibre tracts in one or both temporal lobes without removal of tissue) may help to control the mental state of patients with temporal lobe epilepsy, and has the advantage of producing a minimal neurological deficit.

Aside from patients who have benign cerebral tumours, and who generally improve greatly if the tumour can be completely removed, neurosurgery may play an important role in controlling seizures originating from other gross destructive lesions such as porencephalic cyst formation. As discussed above, surgery may sometimes be useful in recalcitrant temporal lobe epilepsy. When we turn however to surgical relief of seizures not associated with any obvious pathology, even though the seizures appear to be cortical in origin, but arising outside the temporal lobes, we are on much less certain ground. It is difficult to offer helpful advice about this problem at the present time.

SUMMARY

1. Generalised epilepsy

There is no acceptable surgical treatment for generalised epilepsy at the present time.

2. Partial epilepsy

a. **Extracranial.** Removal of the aetiological condition may be possible, e.g., surgical excision of a pancreatic islet cell adenoma in seizures associated with hypoglycaemia.

b. **Intracranial.** Three groups of patients exist:

(i) Surgery obligatory and likely to be attended by excellent results, e.g., removal of a mengioma.

(ii) Surgery likely to be beneficial in selected patient, e.g. cortical cicatrix
porencephalic cyst
arteriovenous malformation
cerebral palsy with hemiplegia and epilepsy.

(iii) Surgery possible but results variable e.g., in temporal lobe epilepsy when there is no obvious lesion and medical treatment has failed.

FURTHER READING

Davidson S, Falconer M A 1975 Outcome of surgery in 40 children with temporal lobe epilepsy. Lancet 2: 1260
Falconer M A 1970 Significance of surgery for temporal lobe epilepsy in children and adolescence. J Neurosurg 33: 233
Rasmussen T, Gossman H 1963 Epilepsy due to gross destructive brain lesions. Neurology (Minneap) 13: 659

10

Prognosis

Mirantur tactiti, et dubio pro fulmine pendent.
(They wonder in silence, and stand in anxious fear as to the uncertain fall of the thunderbolt).

Publius Papinius Statius
61–96 A.D.

The general public remains very ignorant about epilepsy and tends to equate the condition with mental illness. The diagnosis of epilepsy poses problems not only in management but in the education of the patient and his relatives regarding the nature of the illness and the outlook for the future. The physician must therefore have an adequate understanding of the prognosis of the different varieties of epilepsy he may be called upon to diagnose and treat. He will probably be asked 'Does this mean he will become insane?'; or 'Will he outgrow the seizures and stop having attacks?'; or 'Has he a tumour?' In this chapter, some guidance on these and related subjects will be offered.

It has already been emphasised that effective management of epilepsy depends primarily on an accurate and comprehensive diagnosis. The same applies to prognosis, and it is essential that the clinician makes an adequate assessment of the patient before attempting to express an opinion as to the course of future events.

GENERALISED EPILEPSY

Absences (petit mal)
In discussing the prognosis of petit mal absences, it is necessary to emphasise again that in this book the terms 'petit mal' and 'absence' are employed to denote a particular variety of epilepsy characterised clinically by brief absences and electroencephalographically by bursts of bilaterally symmetrical and synchronous 3 Hz spike and slow wave activity (p. 19). Thus, by definition, we exclude minor epileptic events due, for example, to abnormal electrical activity in one or both

temporal lobes. It is also important to distinguish between petit mal absences (and petit mal absences associated with major tonic-clonic seizures) and minor bilateral myoclonic seizures with electro-encephalographic evidence of multiple spikes in addition to the 3 Hz slow wave complexes, or spike and wave complexes at a frequency other than 3 Hz (petit mal variant). The latter are usually due to acquired pathology.

Petit mal absence epilepsy

This is not a particularly common form of epilepsy. It is typically a condition of childhood and there is a tendency for it to cease spontaneously. Thus, some 25 per cent of patients will cease to have absences by 15 years, 50 per cent by 20 years and 75 per cent by 30 years. Indeed, it is uncommon to encounter petit mal absences in adult life although if the absences continue up to the third decade of life they often continue indefinitely. Adults, however, appear to learn to live with absences and disregard them.

Petit mal absence status

One hazard of this type of epilepsy is the development of petit mal status, a condition in which the child becomes inattentive, confused and disorientated for hours on end and, apparently inexplicably, his school work falls well behind his usual performance. In such patients the E.E.G. may show virtually continuous generalised 3 Hz spike and wave activity. Although mental retardation is otherwise extremely uncommon in petit mal, repeated attacks of petit mal status may have an adverse effect on the child's intellectual status and the later development of major seizures is very common.

Petit mal absences with tonic-clonic seizures

Petit mal absence may be associated with major seizures. In such instances the prognosis must be more guarded than that for petit mal alone. Further, in some 50 per cent of patients who have had petit mal for a number of years, major tonic-clonic seizures develop and replace the classical absences as the patient becomes older. There is some evidence to suggest that the subsequent development of tonic-clonic seizures may be minimised if patients presenting with petit mal absences are treated with drugs active against generalised convulsive seizures as well as with drugs to suppress absences. In patients who have, or develop, tonic-clonic seizures as well as petit mal, the prognosis is the same as that for primary generalised epilepsy with tonic-clonic convulsive seizures.

Myoclonic epilepsy

Infantile myoclonic seizures (infantile spasms, hypsarrhythmia) are associated with a substantial risk of permanent intellectual retardation unless the disorder is fully controlled within a few days or weeks of its onset. Even if it is, evidence of an underlying progressive brain disease e.g. tuberose sclerosis, may appear later. Some 50 per cent of cases of hypsarrhythmia have underlying progressive or non-progressive brain pathology. If infantile spasms cannot be controlled the myoclonic seizures ultimately die out, but other forms of epilepsy, often tonic-clonic convulsions, occur and the sufferer commonly proves to have refactory epilepsy and to be mentally backward and virtually unemployable, even if no underlying brain disease is found.

Childhood myoclonic seizures occasionally appear to be of hereditary origin and not associated with underlying structural brain pathology. Such seizures may respond to therapy with, for example, ethosuximide and the long term prognosis may be reasonable. More often childhood myoclonic seizures mount in frequency and severity. In this *Lennox-Gastaut syndrome* the seizures often take the form of drop attacks and their frequency and severity interfere with education. Such seizures are often difficult to control (sodium valproate being the most useful drug.) The myoclonic seizures may or may not diminish in adolescence and early adult life, but the sufferer often develops generalised convulsive seizures and is educationally backward and difficult to employ.

Myoclonic seizures beginning in adolescence are often relatively easy to control with phenobarbitone or one of its congeners. If such seizures remain fully controlled for several years the prospect for permanent cure is reasonably good. However some patients also develop tonic-clonic fits if their myoclonic attacks are not controlled quickly enough. Myoclonic epilepsy in this age group is usually not associated with clinically detectable structural brain pathology. When it is the prognosis is more doubtful.

Tonic-clonic seizures

Perhaps the most benign variety of primarily generalised epilepsy is the so-called *simple febrile convulsion*. This type of epilepsy commences in the first few years of life and in approximately 90 per cent of patients the seizures cease spontaneously by 10 years of age. In some 10 per cent of patients, however, seizures may continue as manifestations of generalised epilepsy or as manifestations of ischaemic cortical damage sustained during the febrile convulsions; in other words, secondary partial epilepsy may become grafted onto the primary generalised type.

A similar group, with an extremely good prognosis, consists of children who have a seizure or a group of seizures in the first few years of life, who show no evidence of brain pathology and who receive early treatment and are rapidly controlled by anticonvulsant therapy. In this group the relapse rate is probably not greater than 15 per cent.

Primary tonic-clonic (grand mal) epilepsy. This usually develops before adult life, sometimes in persons who have had absence or myoclonic seizures, sometimes as the first manifestation of epilepsy. Anticonvulsant drugs are then prescribed and in the majority of instances the seizures are controlled. At this stage, parents should be told that this therapy must be continued, without sudden cessation or interruption, for a minimum period of three to five years and that no firm prognosis can be given as to whether or not the drugs can eventually be withdrawn until this period has elapsed, although there is a reasonable chance that the patient can 'grow out of' the condition. At the end of a three year (or longer) period during which there has been complete control of seizures, the position can be reviewed; if the E.E.G. has become normal it is reasonable to withdraw the anti-convulsant drugs gradually over a period of 6 to 12 months and, provided the patient remains seizure-free, the drugs can then be discontinued. Thereafter, it is quite possible that the patient will remain well and free of seizures; in other patients further attacks may occur in a completely unpredictable manner either soon after the drug is withdrawn, or several years later. In such instances anticonvulsant therapy should be resumed in the previous effective dosage. If, on the other hand the E.E.G. continues to show abnormal activity, it is unlikely that the patient will remain seizure-free if the drugs are withdrawn and a further 12 to 24 months period of drug therapy is generally advisable with further review at the end of this time. If the patient remains seizure-free over a period of four to five years yet the electroencephalo-gram continues to be abnormal, periodic gradual reduction of drug therapy can be attempted.

In general, it can be emphasised that patients with epilepsy generally have many fewer seizures than is popularly supposed; many have only two to three attacks per year. Further, provided reasonable control is achieved, epilepsy does not lead to mental deterioration. However, frequent grand mal seizures may lead to cumulative brain damage and to progressive intellectual deterioration as a result of repeated episodes of cerebral hypoxia.

In some patients suppression of seizures appears to lead to a personality change which is often more trying to parents than an occasional seizure. In this event additional psychotropic drugs may be given. If these are of no avail, it may sometimes be better to allow the child to have a few seizures if this minimises the personality disturbance.

Anticonvulsant drugs may produce undue somnolence, irritability or abnormal behaviour and in some children a deterioration in scholastic status may occur.

Consideration should also be given to the fact that many chronic conditions result in the individual's becoming anxious, depressed or even paranoid.

Finally, sudden withdrawal of anticonvulsants, or impaired absorption due to intercurrent disease such as diarrhoea or vomiting, may lead to the development of status epilepticus.

PARTIAL EPILEPSY

Partial epileptic seizures, with or without secondary generalisation (grand mal), occurring for the first time in adult life, *if unrelated to head injury*, must be regarded as being of serious prognostic significance. In adult patients under the age of 50 years, a cerebral tumour will be responsible for the onset of epilepsy in some 10–15 per cent of patients; in those over 50 years of age, epilepsy will relate to cerebrovascular disease in approximately 60 per cent and to intracranial neoplasms in 25 per cent. Moreover, in patients over 50 years of age there is an increased risk of a metastatic intracranial tumour being responsible. Since tumours superficially situated over the hemispheres, such as meningiomata, are commonly associated with epilepsy, operative removal of the tumour is possible in some 30 to 50 per cent of patients with epilepsy due to a space occupying intracranial lesion.

When partial epilepsy begins in childhood the risk of tumour or other serious underlying brain disease is substantially less than in adults. This risk, however, is not negligible. In particular, the possibility of a cerebral abscess should be considered if the child has a source of infection in the ear, nasal sinuses, lungs or heart, or if there has been a head injury. Most cases of partial epilepsy beginning in childhood are due to brain injury at birth.

When partial epilepsy is due to non-progressive brain pathology it is difficult to know the outlook for cure of the epilepsy till there has been time for a trial of anticonvulsant therapy. In general the earlier in the course of the disorder anticonvulsant treatment is instituted, and the more carefully such therapy is used, the better the prognosis for long term seizure control and ultimate cure. As in managing generalised tonic-clonic epilepsy, complete seizure control should be maintained for three to five years before withdrawal of therapy is contemplated.

Post-traumatic epilepsy. In post-traumatic epilepsy it is possible to offer firmer advice about prognosis than in other varieties of partial epilepsy. An epileptic seizure following within minutes of a relatively minor head injury (*'immediate epilepsy'*) is usually entirely benign and the patient remains well thereafter. The development, however, of epileptic attacks in the week following a significant head injury (*'early epilepsy'*), and particularly if there is a depressed fracture or prolonged post-traumatic amnesia, carries with it an enhanced risk of post-traumatic epilepsy (*'late epilepsy'*) developing in the future (p. 32). If true post-traumatic epilepsy (i.e., 'late epilepsy' or epilepsy developing one week or more after the injury) does develop, the seizures can be controlled by anticonvulsant therapy in the majority of patients and in 50 per cent the seizures will cease spontaneously after a few years. Therefore, as in other forms of epilepsy, a gradual reduction and finally withdrawal of drug therapy after a seizure-free period of three years is warranted. Following a bout of 'early epileptic seizures', there is some evidence to suggest that the exhibition of anticonvulsants (e.g. phenytoin) for a period of 12 to 24 months minimises the risk of 'late epilepsy' developing.

In some patients with resistant post-traumatic epilepsy, operative removal of a cicatrix or resection of an epileptic focus in the wall of a post-traumatic porencephalic cyst may render the patient more responsive to anticonvulsant drug therapy.

EPILEPSY DUE TO EXTRACRANIAL CAUSES

As explained earlier, epilepsy due to extracranial causes may present either as generalised or as partial seizures. In patients whose epileptic seizures are due to extracranial causes, the prognosis is that of the primary pathology. Thus, epilepsy occurring as a complication of eclampsia or delirium tremens will have a good prognosis if the toxaemia condition and the epilepsy are adequately treated. Patients with hypoglycaemia may respond extremely well if the islet cell adenoma is effectively removed (and if the adenoma is single and benign), whereas epilepsy occurring as a complication of uraemia in chronic renal disease will have a correspondingly bad prognosis unless relieved by dialysis or renal transplant. It should also be remembered that if the epileptic seizures in this group of conditions are sufficiently severe or prolonged, secondary cerebral changes from anoxic or hypoglycaemic neuronal damage may result in secondary epilepsy (of intracranial origin) developing as a complication of the primary extracranial disease.

NEONATAL EPILEPSY

It is often difficult to classify neonatal seizures as generalised or partial because of technical difficulties in carrying out adequate electro-encephalography in this age group, and because seizure activity may propogate differently in the very immature brain. Therefore neonatal seizures are discussed separately. The prognosis for children who develop seizures during the neonatal period is often grave, in that the babies frequently die from the gross underlying neurological damage (brain injury with haemorrhage; congenital brain defects; kernicterus; sepsis with cortical thrombophlebitis). In those who survive, however, a considerable proportion may remain seizure-free. Metabolic disturbance e.g. hypoglycaemia, may also cause neonatal seizures. Here, with appropriate treatment, the prognosis is good.

SUMMARY

1. Generalised epilepsy

a. Absences (petit mal)

(i) Petit mal attacks cease by 20 to 30 years in majority of patients.

(ii) Risk of petit mal status and intellectual deterioration.

(iii) Petit mal may be associated with major seizures—prognosis as in 1. c (ii). below

(iv) Petit mal may be replaced by major seizures at puberty or later.

b. Myoclonic attacks

(i) Infantile spasms have a bad prognosis for subsequent epilepsy and mental retardation unless controlled early.

(ii) Lennox-Gastaut syndrome in childhood has a bad prognosis for subsequent epilepsy and backwardness.

(iii) Idiopathic myoclonic epilepsy in adolescence has a good prognosis if adequately treated.

c. Tonic-clonic generalised epilepsy

(i) Febrile convulsions ⎰ 90 per cent of patients
Seizures in first few years of life ⎯ will cease to have
with no evidence of brain damage. ⎱ seizures.

(ii) Tonic-clonic (major) seizures commencing before adult
life.

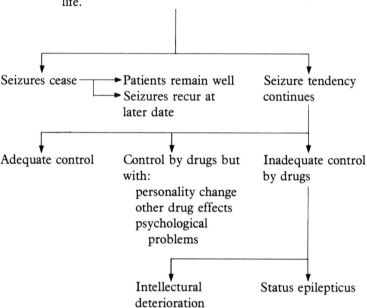

2. Partial epilepsy

a. Partial epilepsy occurring for first time in adult life:
Under 50 years of age: intracranial tumour in 10–15 per cent of
patients.
Over 50 years of age: cerebrovascular disease in 60 per cent;
intracranial tumours in 25 per cent and mestastatic tumours
common.
In patients with intracranial tumour a benign lesion present in
30–50 per cent.

b. Post traumatic epilepsy:
50 per cent cease spontaneously after a few years.
Majority of others controlled by anticonvulsants.
Drug resistant patients may benefit from surgery.

3. Epilepsy due to extracranial causes

Prognosis will depend on underlying disease, for example:
Toxaemia of pregnancy: good.
Islet cell adenoma: Good if single and benign.
Uraemia from chronic renal disease: hopeless without dialysis or
renal transplant.

4. Neonatal seizures

(i) + gross brain damage: bad prognosis.

(ii) + minimal brain damage: seizures may cease.

(iii) due to metabolic disturbance: good prognosis, if treated appropriately.

FURTHER READING

Holowach J, Thurston D L, O'Leary L 1972 Prognosis in childhood epilepsy. Follow-up study of 148 cases in which therapy had been suspended after prolonged anticonvulsant control. New Engl J Med 286: 169

Keith H M 1964 Convulsions in children under three years of age. A study of prognosis. Proc Mayo Clinic 39: 895

Livingston S, Torres I, Pauli L L, Rider R V 1965 Petit mal epilepsy. J Amer Med Ass 194: 227

Rodin E A 1968 The prognosis of patients with epilepsy. Charles C. Thomas, Springfield

Serafetinides E A, Cominian J 1963 A follow up study of late-onset epilepsy. 1. Neurological findings. Brit Med J 1: 428

Sumi S M, Teasdall R D 1963 Focal seizures of review of 150 cases. Neurology (Minneap) K3: 582

Woodcock S, Cosgrove J B R 1964 Epilepsy after the age of 50. Neurology (Minneap) 14: 34

General bibliography

Critchley MacD, O'Leary J L, Jennett B 1972 Scientific foundations of neurology.
William Heinemann, London
Gastaut H, Broughton R 1972 Epileptic seizures. Clinical and electrographic features,
diagnosis and treatment. Charles C. Thomas, Springfield
Laidlaw J P, Richens A 1976 A textbook of epilepsy. Churchill Livingstone, Edinburgh
Magnus O, Lorentz de Hass A M 1974 The epilepsies. In: Vinken P J, Bruyn G W (eds)
Handbook of clinical neurology. North Holland, Amsterdam, vol 15
Magoun H W 1963 The waking brain. 2nd edn Charles C. Thomas, Springfield
Meyer A 1958 Epilepsy. In: Greenfield J G, Blackwood W, McMenemy W H, Meyer A,
Norman R, (eds) Neuropathology. Edward Arnold, London
Neidermeyer E 1974 Compendium of the epilepsies. Charles C. Thomas, Springfield
Penfield W, Jasper H 1954 Epilepsy and the functional anatomy of the human brain.
Little, Brown & Co., Boston
Temkin O 1971 The falling sickness. A history of epilepsy from the Greeks to the
beginning of modern neurology. Johns Hopkins Press, Baltimore
Walter W Grey 1963 The living brain. Duckworth, London

Index